1 MONTH OF
FREE
READING

at

www.ForgottenBooks.com

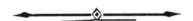

By purchasing this book you are eligible for one month membership to ForgottenBooks.com, giving you unlimited access to our entire collection of over 1,000,000 titles via our web site and mobile apps.

To claim your free month visit:

www.forgottenbooks.com/free870533

ISBN 978-0-266-58252-6
PIBN 10870533

For support please visit www.forgottenbooks.com

UPPER CANADA JOURNAL

OF

𝕸𝖊𝖉𝖎𝖈𝖆𝖑, 𝕾𝖚𝖗𝖌𝖎𝖈𝖆𝖑, 𝖆𝖓𝖉 𝕻𝖍𝖞𝖘𝖎𝖈𝖆𝖑 𝕾𝖈𝖎𝖊𝖓𝖈𝖊.

VOl. 2 8-9

MONTHS—JANUARY AND FEBRUARY—1853.

TORONTO:

PRINTED FOR THE PROPRIETOR BY A. F. PLEES, 113, KING STREET EAST.

1853.

VOL. II   JANUARY AND FEBRUARY, 1853.   NOS. 8 & 9.

CONTENTS:

NOTICE.

The Publisher begs to notify the Medical men, and Naturalists, that he can supply a limited number of copies of Dr Goadby's communication on the Preservation of Animal Substances, in pamphlet form, distinct from the Medical Journal, price 1s. 3d.

The Publisher also informs Dr. Goadby, that notwithstanding the shameful manner in which he broke his engagement, to supply matter for the completion of the promised volume, that a fair proportion of the above copies may be had upon application.

113, King St. East, Toronto, 1853.

THE

UPPER CANADA JOURNAL

OF

𝔐edical, 𝔖urgical, and 𝔓hisical 𝔖cience.

FOR JANUARY AND FEBRUARY, 1853.

ORIGINAL COMMUNICATIONS.

ART. XXVII.—*The Hip Joint, considerations on its injuries and disease, deduced from the Anatomy, by S. J. Stratford M. R. C. S. Eng. Toronto. Continued from the last Journal.*

INFLAMMATION OF THE SYNOVIAL MEMBRANE.

In the last Journal, we endeavoured to present a detail of the anatomy of the Hip-joint, confident that a due appreciation of the various structures will lead us to a just knowledge of its diseases—while an attentive consideration of the action of the various muscles which operate upon the parts, will at a future period, we doubt not, be found clearly to indicate the nature of the accidents; and will teach us a facility of relieving them, especially when displacement has occurred, that will appear very surprising when contrasted with the common modes of proceeding in such cases.—We also entered upon the consideration of inflammation of the synovial membrane of the Hip joint, when we endeavoured to point out the indications of Hyperœmic action — of serous effusion and of the production of false membrane in the joint—and must now proceed to the consideration of the next stages of the disease.

We have shown that from the effusion of the exudation Corpuscles, we have the formation of false membrane, a variety of areola tissue, this is a marked indication of the law of analogous formations.

there is no doubt that the laws of Analagous formation, in the several structures of the body, are obscured with doubt and con_fusion.—It is clear however that the blastema, in which is produced or generated, all the variety of cell formations, both normal and abnormal, is a product of the blood, effused from its vessels—and the question to be decided appears to be, whether the white cor-puscle of the blood escaping with the blastema, that circulates in each different structure, is the true exudation corpuscle—or if within the blastema escaped from each structure, we have a cell nucleus capable of generating its like in the new formation. The strict conformity of some morbid products, such as pus, which is the same in every variety of structure, would lead us to believe that the difference consisted in a change of the exudation corpuscle rather than the escape of these cell-nuclei, for if such was the case, these must exist in the blood of every individual structure as a primary element perceptible to the microscope—this is not con-sistent with the fact,for the blastema was but a few moments before, part of the Liquor Sanguinis passing to, and indiscriminately nourishing all the normal structures of the body without giving rise to any such formation as pus.

There is one fact which may in some degree serve to explain the difference of Pathologists respecting the formation of the pus-corpuscle, from, the white globules of the blood, is that these, with a good microscope may be seen to be of various sizes in the normal condition, hence in the Liquor puris, we should expect to find pus-corpuscles in different stages of development, consonant with this curious fact—and so we find them.

Suppose the disease should still progress, the arterial excite-ment already spread to the other textures of the joint—these now participate in the inflammatory action. If it has extended to the capsular ligament, the amount of pain is greatly increased, and its nature is considerably changed, it is the dull sickening ache of the fibrous tissues ; could we observe the appearance of the ligament it would be seen of a pink colour, like the selerotic coat of the eye, for now its capillary vessels carry red blood. So also will the cartilages of the Joint participate in the Hyperœmic action, the vascular structure from which it receives nourishment, becomes distended with a denser fluid, that causes the fibrous portion of its structure to swell, fills its cells to their utmost extent, and may be one of the principal causes of the elongation of the thigh in acute inflammation of the Hip Joint. The inflammatory fever is now extreme, the pain also becomes insufferable, so that the least movement of the joint causes excruciating suffering, and the patient instinctively and rigidly maintains one position, he cannot bear even the least change of his pillow, even the rude walking of people upon the floor, increases his irritability if not his actual torture, and he pertinaceously lies in all the filthiness of a sick bed. This condition of things is doubtless a provision of nature, to pre-esrve the most profound rest to the joint, for in this case motion would do the greatest harm, it would increase the inflammatory action, and assist to develop the formation of matter in the joint, a point when it has happened, from which we shall have to date changes of the most formidable character, and which in our opinion must ever after be associated with lameness, and deformity.

The disease may now stop short of the actual development of the pus globule, as I have shown the plastic lymph may have taken on a healthy action, may have become organized, but the joint remains swelled, stiff, and attended with considerable lameness, which subsides but by slow degrees; should now however the presumptuous Quack, interfere with this process of nature (which I have known to occur) and dare to twist and turn the limb, under pretext of reducing luxation of the joint, I need not picure the dreadful intensity of the patient's suffering, or show the enormity of the act, which will in all probability hurry the disease o a fatal termination, whereby perpetual lameness and deformity, f not actual death is the result. This state and condition of the oint, is not unfrequently caused by falls upon the trochanter major, whereby the head of the bone is violently driven into the cetabulum—the delicate synovial apparatus of the joint is injured, nd more or less inflammatory action of this structure is the esult.

Should the progress of the disease continue, the plastic cytolastema effused into the joint and surrounding tissues, begins to often, the formation of the pus-corpuscle now happens, and mater rapidly accumulates in the joint. The advent of this eriod is generally marked by rigours of more or less severity which seize the patient in token of the alarm the constitution now els, for the vast importance of this stage of the disease—the us thus formed in the joint, is developed from the effused lymph hich has been described as one of the results of congestive tion, in the vessels of the synovial membrane, during a state inflammation; this instead of becoming organized, and remainng a permanent false membrane in the joint, the effused plasma oner or later begins to soften, and we observe corpuscles to be med in the dissolved fibrine, these floating in the Liquor puris, the pus-corpuscles.—The perfectl formed pus-corpuscles are ls containing one or more nuclei, metimes even nucleoli. us we may observe a simple and app ently vesicular nucleus, ced excentrically in a transparent elast and round cell-wall; a subsequent period the nucleus see to have a granular,

amorphose precipitate around it, without a clear outer circumference; upon an attentive examination we can also observe in the
fluid minute granules less than the 1000th of an inch in diameter,
while larger corpuscles identical with the nuclei of pus-corpuscle are observable. The history of the process would lead to the
belief that two or three of these nuclei may be grouped together,
in all probability and to all appearance exudation corpuscles, these
having taken on a required action and having a cell-wall developed
around them at first pale and transparent, but subsequently becoming thickened opaque and covered with granules—hence the various structures visible by a microscope, observed floating in the
Liquor Puris—the progress of this process in the development of
the pus-corpuscles, is often extremely rapid, a few hours sufficing
to exhibit a full grown corpuscle; as soon as the cell-wall is formed
the corpuscle grows by endosmotic action, and after a time having
ran through its course, it bursts, and liberates the granules, which
are often all that can be found in the pus that has been evacuated
from the body after several days.

The joint now soon becomes greatly distended with pus, so much
so, that ulceration of the synovial membrane, and also of the Capsular Ligaments will take place, from the great distension of the
part, when the patient experiences a temporary relief from the pain
—by degrees the pus escaping among the muscles of the hip,
burrows down in every direction, until it finds its way to the surface; and this may show itself near the groin, or on the back of
the hip, while sometimes the abscess will be found to open a long
way down the thigh. Coincident with the formation of matter in
the joint, we find a change in the character of the constitutional
irritation; up to this period the fever has been more or less of the
inflammatory type, the pulse has been full and quick, the tongue
white and loaded, the skin hot and dry, but now the shivering,
which but too plainly marked the baneful change in the nature of
the disease, is frequently repeated, it is followed by heat, and
flushings, and is succeeded by profuse perspiration; the change indicative of this variety of constitutional irritation, returns with more
or less constancy, while the pulse has an enduring frequency, is
small and sharp; a gradual wasting of the body and a progressive
debility of the whole frame, distinctly points out to us the nature
of the change, which has happened in the character of the disease
of the Hip-Joint.

The discharge from the joint is generally in the first instance
normal puss (pus bonum et laudabile) a creamy looking, thick
opaque, and homogenous fluid, having a faint yellowish, sometimes
a white, or even greenish tinge, it has a peculiar smell when fresh,
but looses it on standing, has a sweet mawkish taste, and is

specifically heavier than water—when first evacuated it has an alkaline reaction, but after standing, changes by degrees, so as to exhibit an acid condition; this character of the discharge continues for a longer or shorter period, in all probability dependent upon the amount and rapidity of softening, of the effused blastema, but by degrees the pus looses its normal character, it ceases to be thick and opaque, but becomes thin and transparent, often has an offensive smell, and not unfrequently appears peculiarly acrid and irritating. It now appears evident that a state of transition is progressing; the cells in the amorphose blastema, have become to a considerable extent exhausted, and now the structures of the joint itself are submitted to the dissolving influence of the discharge, are more or less destroyed, and by such means are removed from the system, so that perhaps destruction of the Synovial membrane has become general, ulceration of the cartilages to a considerable extent may have taken place, and the disease have progressed in the bony structure itself until we find that the neck of the thigh bone, and a very considerable part of the cotyloid cavity has been removed from the joint. Consequent upon this destruction and removal of these portions of the joint, we find a great change to occur, for instead of the head of the thigh bone, placed upon its long neck descending into the deep and firm cavity of the acetabulum, having so secure and strong a hold as almost to bid defiance to our attempts at removal, and that even after the tough capsular ligament has been entirely cut through, we find what remains of the head and neck of the bone, protruded from the now comparatively shallow cavity in the bones of the pelvis; in fact the very character of the joint has been changed by the disease, so that the natural action of the muscles which perform its several movements in a normal condition, are now able to produce a separation of the bones; all the natural continuity, between the femur and colyloid cavity being dissolved, dislocation of the hip joint is the consequence. The direction in which this dislocated extremity of the thigh bone shall be placed, would seem to be dependent upon the position of the limb at the moment of this separation, if the patient lying upon his back in bed, should have flexed the knee, adducted the thigh, and have rotated the toe inwards, so as to have relieved the surface of the joint from all pressure in the first instance, and have subsequently maintained that position inflexibly, as soon as the disease shall have so far progressed that the joint shall cease to offer the natural impediments to the retraction of the thigh bone this will be drawn upwards by the action of the great muscles, and lodged upon dorsum of the Illium ; again the position of the patient may have become changed from the weariness of his posture, should he have turned upon his side, and thereby have abducted the flexed thigh, the bone may be located in the thyroid hole ; it may bé placed in any position in which the action of the muscles shall be favoured by the position of the bone at the moment of separation ; this may perhaps account for the striking varieties we find in the deformities dependent upon this disease.

This separation of the diseased surfaces of the joint, would appear to be a provision of nature, towards the cure of this complaint; the diseased structures now comparatively cease to be a source of mutual irritation, and the patient often dates the favourable changes in the diseased action, from this period of time. As soon as the dislocation of the thigh bone upon the dorsum of the Ilium has been produced, considerable shortening of the limb is the result, the knee is bent and the foot rotated inwards ; that the amount of this inversion (which varies with the circumstances of each case) will depend upon the length of the neck of the thigh bone that remains attached to the shaft; if this be considerable the action of the rotator muscles of the hip arising from the pelvis, and inserted into the trochanter major, will bind the shaft firmly to the pelvis, while the extended neck preventing the rotatory action of these muscles, will be found to preserve the limb in the one position ; but should the neck have been wholly removed by the diseased action, the rotatory movement of the shaft will be permitted; and we may even find a complete evertion of the foot, should the bone when removed from the colyloid cavity, have been placed in the thyroid hole, the limb will be somewhat lengthened, the thigh abducted and the toe turned outwards—As the patient gains his strength and assumes the erect posture, the change in the position of femur will cause an alteration in the line of the pelvis, and as a necessary consequence of this condition, a sigmoid flexure of the spine is the result —according to the amount of the inclination of the pelvis from its normal position, will be the amount of this curvature of the spine. In dislocation upwards the pelvis is inclined to the diseased side, to enable the shortened limb to rest upon the ground, the vertical condition of the vertebral column is deranged, and flexon in an opposite direction is the necessary result; no sooner has this been accomplished than the body is thrown too far on the opposite side, and to gain the true perpendicular, so that the head may rest perfectly on the top of the column, and be truly balanced in the centre of gravity, that another curve is necessary, but this is scarcely more than half the dimensions of the former —hence the characteristic sigmoid flexure of the spine. This condition has equally an effect, if the limb is lengthened by being placed in the thyroid hole, but exactly in the reversed direction.

I have already pointed out, that the formation of matter in

the joint, has been followed by ulceration of the capsular ligament, and the escape of the pus without the shut sack—that it
burrows in many directions, undermining the parts about the joint,
isolating the muscles from their connection with the bones, causing
extensive disease of the bones of the pelvis, or having extended
among the muscles of the hip it will destroy the fascia, and leave
very extensive sinuses—moreover the disease may extend by ulceration, (especially in young subjects) through the bottom of the
colyloid cavity, insinuate itself under the Illiac muscle within the
pelvis, and has even been known to cause adhesions and disease
of the large intestine in its immediate vicinity, so that the matter
in the diseased hip-joint has been evacuated through the
bowels.

This state of things may have continued for a longer or shorter period, often in young people the progress of this disease may
be very rapid, may have caused intense constitutional irritation
that was attended with violent delirium or continued hectic, accompanied with profuse sweating; may have so debilitated the
patient that the powers of his constitution sink, and death closes
the scene.　But if on the separation of the diseased bones, or from
some other favourable cause, the diseased action should take a
more fortunate turn, the great purulent discharge begins to
subside, the sinuses to heal up, and the patient's constitution to
regain a degree of tone and elasticity, the harbinger of returning
health.　The bone now begins to be accustomed to its new situation among the muscles of the hip, exostosis occurs to a certain
extent, often very considerable, it surrounds the extremity of
the femur, and after a time accomplishes the formation of a new
cavity, giving rise to the production of a new joint—in whatsoever
part the femur shall be located, whether it be on the dorsum of the
Illium, the thyroid hole, or in any other situation.　Sometimes the
shaft of the thigh bone becomes firmly adherent in the new formation, and fixed in one position, often not the most advantageous,
and although it is fully able to bear the weight of the body in its
new position, it is not permited the least latitude of motion—it is an
anchylosed joint.　The Colyloid cavity also becomes completely
filled with a new formation of bone, and the result of the heal-
hy action, is the total subsidence of the disease, a cure, which
under the most favourable circumstances however, is but an alter-
nation between death and deformity.

Such is the course of the inflammation of the synovial membrane of the hip joint, that after a time has evidently extended to all
the other structures, implicating them in changes of the most
grave description ; doubtless every case will exhibit a shade of
difference either in the intensity of its symptoms, or the character

of its existing cause.   In some cases preeminently acute, the symptoms will be extremely rapid, will evince all the characters of intense inflammatory action, and may arrive at a fatal termination in the short space of a week or ten days; but in the generality of cases the progress of the disease will be much more tardy.   It may come on with scarcely an indication of its approach, by the sudden appearance of swelling of the joint attended with acute pain caused by any active exertion ; it may have as suddenly subsided, without any permanent ill effects, to be reexcited however upon the application of any other exciting cause, or the advent of any inflammatory condition of the constitution, which will predispose to such diseases.

In the knee the swelling and effusion, which so rapidly occurs, in inflammation of the synovial membrane, is easily recognized, and truly forms a most characteristic feature in the complaint, although equally present in this disease when occurring in the hip-joint, but from the greater depth of the cotyloid cavity, is far less easily recognized, but even here it may be observed upon due and attentive consideration.   It must however be confessed that the inflammatory action in this disease will extend so rapidly to the other structures of the joint, as speedily to obscure this distinctive symptom, as in its progress it involves the other structures of the joint; while itself becomes a frequent accompaniment of other diseases, developed during their progress, and this is especially the case, in inflammation of the Capsular Ligaments of the joint, on which it is a pretty constant attendant.

It is to be observed that the rapidity with which the symptoms of this disease generally progress, are the most distinctive characteristic of inflammation of the synovial membrane—the acute pain and rapid swelling, serve to mark the distinction from chronic inflammation of the cartilage, and that variety of irritation which proceeds from deposition of tubercular matter in the several structures of the hip-joint; while the character of the pain, and the constitutional pecularities, serve to distinguish it from inflammation of the Ligamenteous textures.

To be continued.

[Errata in last number, page 207, line 2, for pernation read hœmatin.]

Art. XXVIII.—*A Practical Treaties on the Art of making and Preserving Microscopical and other Preparations.*   By Henry Goadby, M.D., F.L.S.

In the preserving fluids that I use, and which are known by my name, the following ingredients occur, viz. : rock salt, alum, corrosive sublimate, and the white oxyd of arsenic, or arsenious acid.

These materials are never all employed at one time, and they should be used judiciously, to prevent the contingency of destroying rather than preserving specimens of Natural History.

To this end, I think it desirable to describe the *properties* of the materials respectively, before giving the necessary formulæ for the fluids.

Rock (or bay) salt is very preservative, and will maintain the characteristics of all tissues unimpaired, better than any other agent with which I am acquainted, provided the *strength* be well regulated ; and I make much greater use of the purely saline, or B fluid, than of any other.

Alum possesses very important conservative properties ; it is astringent, coagulates albumen to some extent, rendering transparent tissues opake in proportion to the volume of alum brought in contact with them ; but it *destroys the carbonate of lime,* converting it into the insoluble sulphate. The aluminous, or A, 2, fluid, however, is a very valuable composition ; and to it I owe many important preparations, which may be found both in my own possession, and in the Hunterian Museum of the Royal College of Surgeons, of England, and which never could have been made without its assistance.

Alum *combines* with animal tissues so perfectly, that it cannot be dissolved out of them by long continued maceration in water. Whenever it is considered necessary to use the aluminous fluids either to give form, and support, to an animal, or any part of an animal, or a delicate tissue, by reason of its astringent property, or to render diaphanous animals or tissues opake enough to be visible, *the excess of alum* should be washed away with water, and the animal, or whatever it might be, with few exceptions, removed from the aluminous, and preserved permanently in the B fluid. It should be constantly borne in mind that the effect of fresh volumnes of the aluminous fluid should be cautiously watched, lest the alum produce mischievous results; but with care it may even be used to the full extent of its valuable properties on the soft parts of an animal enclosed in a shell of carbonic of lime, or oth-wise possessing that earth, for the muscular, nervous, and other soft tissues, will be much sooner affected by the action of the alum than the denser tissues containing earthy matter. It will hence be seen that the aluminous fluid is not of universal application.

Corrosive sublimate is also astringent, and the coagulator of albumen; the intention of its application is not for the sake of either of these properties, but simply to prevent vegetation *growing in the fluids* respectively. But inasmuch as albumen takes from corrosive sublimate a portion of its chlorine, and thus converts it into calomel, and as all animal tissues are more or less albuminous, the propriety of using it at all, may well be questioned. In places where the sporules of fungi abound, as in the store-rooms of large museums, not even the presence of corrosive sublimate can prevent them from *growing upon the surface of either* of my preserving fluids, if they contain animal matter of any kind and are in *open* vessels, i. e., not hermetically sealed; but in a long experience of this fact, I am bound to say, although I have had open jars, dishes, and other vessels containing dissections of animals waiting their turn to be mounted permanently as preparations, in which the surface of the fluid has been covered during the summer months with vegetation of considerable substance, and which has continued to increase, and flourish magnificently for weeks, yet, I have never known it to descend into the fluid, or affect the dissections (provided they were well covered with fluid) in any way. Indeed either of these fluids will preserve plants, as easily, and certainly, as they preserve animals; and were the fungus to grow *into* the fluid, it would die, and be preserved, neither have I at any time, during fourteen years experience of preparations made by the use of my fluids, and contained, and sealed down, in the several forms of vessels and cells, also of my invention, ever found a particle of vegetation in a single preparation; and during the last six years I have been using the fluids, both for permanent preparations, and stores, without the addition of corrosive sublimate, and always with satisfactory results.   I believe, therefore, that the corrosive sublimate may be safely left out, although I shall include it in the receipts of the fluids.

Arsenic possesses the power of softening animal tissues to a remarkable extent, and this property has no limit.

A few years ago I was desired by the Examiners in Anatomy, of the University of London, to preserve a body during the summer season for their examinations in the autumn.   Desiring to retain the tissues severally in as natural a state as possible, I added arsenic to the B fluid.   For some months nothing could exceed the success of this experiment, and if I had changed the fluid and substituted B fluid without arsenic, I believe the body would have been permanently preserved.   It was neglected however, in this respect, although I watched it with some solicitude until, after the lapse of rather more than twelve months, I found the entire body (with the exception of the bones) reduced to the condition and appearance of decomposing size, except that it remained perfectly sweet.   I have made a number of experiments with the like results. I have seen the characters of muscle, tendon, nerve, &c., gradually disappearing, until nothing but a glairy fluid remained, but was always perfectly sweet.   As arsenic acts upon glass, and glass vessels, by combining with the lead, and for the above reasons, it cannot be employed for preparations that are desired to be permanent.   I have made a few such attempts, but they have all ended in failure.

The softening property is that for which I employ arsenic: either to recover animals that have been hardened, and corrugated in alcohol, or to enable me to proceed with elaborate dissections of nerves which must necessarily be tedious.   My friend Dr. T. S. Beck of London could never have made such a display of the nerves of the uterus—the finest dissection of nerves in the human subject that I believe has ever been made—without the aid of arsenic, which was never allowed to do any mischief, occasionally washed away, then renewed, and so on; and the nerves, under its well regulated influence were as tough as copper wire, and although very delicate in appearance, would bear pulling and stretching with impunity.

The alluminous fluids I originally designated by the letter A, and I called them 1, or 2, as the same weight of the ingredients were dissolved, either in one quart of water or two quarts; they are thus made.

A, 2

Rock salt, ...	4 ounces.
Alum, ...	2 ounces.
Corrosive sublimate, . . .	4 grains.
Boiling water, ...	2 quarts.*

The A 1 only differs from the above in having half the quantity of corrosive sublimate, and water. It is very rarely used, being generally too astringent.

B

Rock salt, ...	8 ounces.
Corrosive sublimate, . . .	2 grains.
Boiling water, ...	1 quart.

The corrosive sublimate must never exceed, under any circumstances, two grains per quart of water; otherwise there will be in time a white precipitate on the preparation that cannot be removed, and which will greatly disfigure it.

When the B fluid is made according to the above receipt, its specific gravity at a temperature of 60 ° will be 1,100, and with it, terrestial and fresh water-animals can be well preserved. In cases where it is desired to preserve the *redness* of muscle, it is only necessary to add the nitrate of potash to the preserving fluid : about half an ounce per quart of fluid.

For marine animals the strength of the fluid must be increased by the addition of salt to 1.148, otherwise they will be decomposed. A great number of marine animals in the first stages of the preserving process require alum, but it must be cautiously used, and carefully watched, and as soon as it has done all that is required of it, the animal should be well washed in clean water and placed in the B fluid. There is no objection to frequent contact with alum, if necessary, provided the process be conducted on the principle here laid down.

---

* The *imperial quart* of 40 ounces is intended to be understood throughout the paper, and the weight, avoirdupoise.

The Arsenical Fluid.—When I employ arsenic for its *soften-ing* properties, I use it alone, unless the process is likely to oc-cupy much time, and in that case, I combine it with the B fluid, in the following proportions, and call it C : B fluid, as di-rected above, arsenic 20 grains. Arsenic can no more be trusted with carbonate of lime, than alum; and if it be desired to employ it on any molluscous animal the creature should be removed from its shell prior to its introduction to arsenic. The solutions of arsenic that I have employed differ in strength from 20 grains to 60 grains to a pint of water, (imperial measure, 20 ounces) or to the pint of B fluid. It is not easy to dissolve this mineral, and the only plan which I have found successful, is to place the quan-tity of arsenic to be dissolved in a Florence oil flask with half a pint of water, apply a spirit lamp, and boil till the whole be dissolved, it can then be diluted by the addition, either of more water, or preserving fluid. I may mention one singular fact of preservation by this fluid, no less of the animal, than (which is most important) its color.

Upwards of six years ago my Son collected for me several specimens of the larvæ of Cossus Ligniperda, the peculiar color of which had never been preserved. In alcoholic fluid, of any strength, it turns quite black, which is a common result of the application of spirit for preserving caterpillars ; in addition, most insect colors are soluble in alcohol.

The specimens included larvæ of the first and second year, and one fine sample of a three-year larva about to turn to a chrysalis. Of the former specimens I preserved some in the A 2, and the rest in the B fluid, and placed the last in a solution of arsenic. The aluminous fluid has hardened and disfigured the caterpillars nearly as much as spirit would have done ; they are softer, and in better state for dissecting, in the B fluid ; but they have lost all their rosy redness of color in both fluids, and are partially black.

It was reserved for the arsenic to give me one caterpillar so beautifully preserved that all its characteristic color, even to the most delicate tint, is maintained to this time. I *believe* that the in-terior has not been destroyed by the softening tendency of arsenic

before alluded to, because, if so, I think there would be con
siderable deposit in the fluid, which has not occurred; neither in
that case would the insect retain its roundness, and fullness, but
on the contrary become flaccid by the removal of those tissues
(muscles) that give form to the integument. As this caterpillar
had been secluded from the operation of light (the fruitful agent
for destroying color in animals) for more than twelve months, I
determined to try the effect of constant exposure, to which I submitted it for three years in England, and for six months in this
country; its beauty is still unimpaired. As it was a sole specimen, and I am not likely to obtain another, I am unwilling to
dissect it.

I have been particular in speaking of the successful application of arsenic in the preservation of *color* in this caterpillar,
because I believe it is of some importance. It is most interesting
to collect the larvæ of Lepidopterous and other insects, as far as
possible, but they lose much value for the purpose of instruction
and for collections, unless their color can be permanently preserved; and I have great hopes that the fluid which has proved
so eminently successful in the instance of the caterpillar of the
goatmoth, which takes on the described blackness a very few
days after death, in every other perserving fluid, may be equally
efficacious in the preservation of color, in the other species.

Mode of using the Preserving Fluids.—A knowledge of the
proper method of using these fluids is essential to success, for in
other hands than my own, they have led to the destruction rather
than the preservation of specimens. Men have constantly treated
my preserving fluids as though they were using spirit, entirely
overlooking one very important consideration, namely, the vast
difference between their specific gravity and that of alcohol. In
the latter, we have a fluid so light that every animal is *heavier,*
and will instantly sink in it; the conditions are exactly reversed
in the former case, where every animal, from an animalcule to
an elephant, is lighter, and will float upon either of them.

Neither of my fluids (always excepting the arsenical) *can be
employed of full strength in the first instance,* and anything to be
preserved in them should undergo previous maceration in clean

cold water, to which, after a time, preserving fluid may be added until the animal rises to the surface. The fluid and the water must be intimately mixed mechanically, or the water will rise through the denser fluid, and retain its integrity for a long time.

The animal will insensibly absorb, and become saturated with the *ingredients* of the preserving fluid, but in a state of considerable dilution ; the strength of the fluid must now be gradually increased, and intimately mixed, until the animal again rise, and in time it will become saturated with this denser fluid. In many instances, it is advisable to keep the animal forcibly at the bottom of the vessel in which it is being preserved *by weights*, and this is particularly necessary in hot weather when the preserving process should be expedited with all the speed that is consistent with safety. It is easy to ascertain if the animal be saturated with the fluid by removing the weights, and in that case, to go on increasing the strength of the fluid : in fine, success depends on carying out the laws of endosmose and exosmose. The diluted fluid used in the first stages should be thrown away, and frequently renewed, as, being replete with animal fluids, it contains within itself the elements of decomposition, and increases the difficulty of obtaining success. This remark, however, applies less to the aluminous, than to the B fluid, as in the former, the coloring matter, and animal deposits of all kinds so abundantly seen when spirit is used and which occasions the steady and constant discoloration of that fluid, for, in some cases, many years, and which so generally tends to the disfigurement of preparations in museums is altogether *insoluble*, from the instant it or they come in contact with alum ; and for this very important reason alum may be almost *always* used in the early stage of preservation, the former cautions on this subject being strictly attended to. Preservation of animals by means of these fluids, then, can only be accomplished by the daily addition of fluid until the creature be saturated with the fluid of the full strength indicated. Nor should the solicitude of the operator end immediately at this point, as it will be necessary occasionally to renew the fluid and often to test its strength. To shorten this species of labor, I long ago procured a glass jar, or tube, two and a half inches long, and three-fourths of an inch wide, with a flat bottom, to be used as a proof-glass ; I then adjusted some specific gravity bubbles so accurately that they *rise very slowly* in the fluid, the precise strength of which they are intended to indicate; if the fluid be weaker than exact strength, they fall to the bottom, and there remain; if stronger, they quickly rise. They are marked on the top A 1, A 2, B, S, the latter indicating a *saturated* solution of rock salt with which it is convenient to increase the daily strength of the B fluid in the manner already described.

By pouring a little fluid into the small proof glass, and applying a bubble as the test of strength of the fluid that has been employed, the operator will instantly learn, not the exact strength, (which is unnecessary,) but that the fluid is either *the* strength, or weaker or stronger; all the information he needs to guide him in his labors.

Instead of the bubble marked " B " I would substitute two, one indicating 1.100 the other 1.148 and the Italian barometer makers could easily graduate such bubbles. The whole apparatus is enclosed in a japanned tin box 1 inch deep, $1\frac{1}{2}$ wide, and $2\frac{7}{8}$ths long, which can be carried in the waiscoat pocket, and costs but little.

When either of the foregoing fluids are required for the display of preparations in a public or private collection, they should be *well filtered*, and for this purpose they may be passed a great number of times through fine flannel rammed into the nozzle of a large earthen funnel, or once through a filtering machine, or twice or thrice through good filter paper. If the filtration be properly performed, these fluids are remarkably bright, white, and brilliant, far exceeding in this respect any alcoholic fluids. Rough filtration may be satisfactorily effected by once passing through the thick flannel used for a jelly bag; but if this be not at hand, it is only necessary to allow the fluids to stand quietly in the vessel in which they were made until quite cold, then carefully pouring off the top, the extraneous matter always found in rock salt will gravitate, especially in the aluminous fluid, which has the property of throwing down any thing which disturbes the transparency of water. Neither of my fluids can be retained in open vessels, glass jars, or even stoppered bottles, for any length of time, without additional protection,

In *open* vessels, the water evaporates, and the salt crystallizes to the total destruction of the specimens included. Salt being highly deliquescent, the volume exposed to atmospheric influence (the upper portion) becomes more or less diluted when the atmosphere contains moisture, and ascends into the neck of the bottle, even around a well ground stopper, by capillary attraction; it gains the upper surface of the stopper and then descends the sides of the bottle, and will lie as a pool on the shelf on which the bottle stands.

As the weather changes, and becomes dry, the salt crystallizes, and thus forms a conduit for the fluid the next rainy day, by which it can greatly, and readily, extend its outposts ; and by this means, in time, it will pass completely out of the bottle or other vessel. Bladder will not confine it, applied to a glass jar on the plan employed for spirit preparations; and the only plan is to cover the jar with a plate of *flat* glass (patent British plate manufactured by Messrs. Chance of Burmingham, is the best) and seal it down with the patent marine glue, applied to the glass, with a hot iron.

The best, neatest, and readiest mode, in my experience is the plan of my invention, namely : first place in the upper vessel of a small copper glue pot some marine glue cut small ; in the lower vessel, where the carpenter would put water, for the careful dissolution of animal glue, put linseed oil, and then apply heat ; the temperature of the boiling oil will dissolve the glue the first, second, and even a third time, with care ; after this it becomes altered in its proportion, and refractory.

The dissolved glue should be rapidly aplied to the rim of the glass jar (which must be quite dry and free from grease,) with a brush, and the only brush that will stand, 1 make in this way. I take a piece of rattan cane as long as a cedar drawing pencil, and cut off the cortex carefully from one end of it to the length I desire the brush to to, being particular not to let the knife go into the substance of the cane any more than I can help. I macerate the prepared end of the cane for a short time in water, and then, while yet wet, I pound it with a hammer upon some hard substance (iron or stone) constantly turning it with my hand until all the fibres of the cane be liberated, and my brush

is complete. I still use a brush of this kind which I have employed for several years extensively, and none other will stand
twice using, the hairs come out with the glue, and are in the
way of a good joint. A disc of glass should be cut to fit the top
of the jar, made clean, and the part that is to be in contact with
the jar also thinly coated with the hot glue. The disc should
previously have had a small hole drilled through the centre,
(about one-eight of an inch in diameter) for a reason that will
presently appear.

The two surfaces of glass being *apparently* [coated with
marine glue, but *really without contact*, the latter must be insured
by means of a hot iron which should be carefully passed over
the surface of the glue several times till it and the glass become
hot, care being taken to keep the iron constantly in motion, and
always on the edge of the jar, or of the disc, as in that case the
expansion will be equal, and no danger occur even if the iron be
red hot; but, it will instantly break if the iron be allowed to
linger in one place, or touch any but the outer portion of the disc,
or rim of the jar.

The jar should be thus prepared while *empty, and dry,* and
when complete, the fluid may be poured in, to about one-half
the height of the jar, together with the preparation to be suspended
in it. The strings necessary for this purpose may be brought
over the edge of the jar, and pressed into the glue on the surface,
if soft enough to admit of it; the preparation may now be regulated
to the required height in the jar, and the threads of suspension
kept in their place by a wet string passed round them on the outside of the jar, several times, and tied. If any fluid chance to be
on the surface of the marine glue on the rim of the jar, it should be
removed; and when dry, the prepared surface of the disc should
be placed on the jar and the two brought together in intimate
contact by the hot iron, which as in the former case, must be
constantly passed round on the edge, and the disc simultaneously
pressed down, until the process be completed. The extraneous
glue on the outer edge may be made smooth and neat, by the
hot iron.

By means of a syringe, to which a small pipe is affixed, fill
up the jar with the preserving fluid, not quite full, however, as

the great expansion of the fluid, (the B. especially) in sudden increase of temperature, may cause the breakage of the top glass; then cut a cork to fit the small hole tightly, insert it, pare it off level with the surface, place upon it a piece of solid marine glue made to adhere to the cork by means of the point of the hot iron, and cover it with another disc of glass about the size of a ten cent piece, or an English six-pence, and the preparation is finished.

It is a good practice to prepare the portion of thread that is to come outside of the jar, the cork, and the surfaces of glass to be coated, with a solution of the marine glue, which may be made by dissolving a piece of glue in an excess of white-wood Naphtha.

Should a stopper become fixed in the neck of a bottle by the crystallization of the salt, it may be easily removed by dissolving the salt by water, and gently tapping the cross piece of the stopper at its extreme ends, (*never across its shorter diameter,*) with a door key. If the cross piece come off, make it and the remainder of the stopper that is in the neck of the bottle hot with the iron, apply marine glue, and cement them together,—when cold, renew your operations,—the stopper is stronger now than before, and will easily come out, and last longer than one not broken. To keep the fluids in stoppered bottles, and to prevent the possibility of the salt crystallizing on the outside of the stopper, the marine glue may be advantageously employed; or a cement, proposed by Prof. Olmsted, of Yale College, and made by melting resin and lard together by the application of heat, and intimately mixing them. The respective quantities of the materials will depend on whether the cement is required to become hard, or not. If the former, the resin must be in excess; if the latter, use more lard. For the purpose that I indicate above, it should be *stiff* and *ropy;* remaining just soft enough in hot weather to spread with a pallette knife.

As a final remark I would say, that the preservation of animals, either in alcoholic, or my fluids, is greatly facilitated by employing, in the first stages of the process, a large volume of fluid.

Crowding animals together in a limited space, and with only a small quantity of fluid, is a fruitful source of injury and loss of the majority, if not of all the specimens; when, however, the preservation is completely effected, the specimens may be packed very closely, together, in a small vessel, and as much fluid of the required strength as will occupy the interstices is amply sufficient for transportation, or stores, and will last for years, especially if the fluid be kept in, by running some marine glue round the stopper and neck of the bottle with a hot iron, or by using the resinous cement.

INSTRUCTIONS FOR MAKING WET PREPARATIONS OF ANIMAL SUBSTANCES.

It frequently happens to the Naturalist, and the Microscopic observer, to meet with animals, or tissues, which, from a variety of circumstances, cannot be retained in any other form than that of a *permanent preparation.* They may be small, and so delicate, that they would be entirely lost if put into a bottle; and in such a case, it is desirable to mount them, without delay, as preparations for the microscope.

If the object be merely a filmy tissue, take a piece of glass of good quality, good surface, and flat; the substance is not material.* Clean it with liquor potassæ or dilute sulphuric acid, or use both these fluids, mixing them on the glass; they effervesce, decompose each other, and at that moment, clean the glass; rinse it in clean soft water and dry it with either a clean muslin hankerchief, or a piece of chamois leather; now test it with a drop of water placed on the centre of one side of the glass, and if the water can diffuse itself *evenly over the whole surface, the glass is clean;* if not, it must be made so.†

This, which is frequently the most difficult part of the whole process, being accomplished, place the glass in the vessel in which the tissue to be mounted lies in preserving fluid, and float it on to the glass; withdraw the latter carefully from the vessel.

---

* The best glass for this purpose is the " patent British plate," manufactured by Messrs. Chance at Birmingham.

† It sometimes happens that neither acid, nor potash can clean a piece of glass sufficiently well to enable it to endure the test proposed; in such a case watery solution of gum arabic may be used, or what is still better—the human saliva will clean it instantly.

With a fine (needle) point adjust the tissue to the centre of the glass, and soak up the excess of fluid with a camel's hair pencil, leaving enough to cover the preparation. Now take a piece of *thin* glass, such as is used by microscopists, previously cut of less width than the slide or glass on which the tissue lies, and having cleaned it by the mode described, hold it at one end by a pair of finely pointed forceps, and apply the outer extremity, holding it almost vertically, to such portion of the other glass as to leave the preparation in the centre of both.

Gradually lower the top glass, and the fluid will run before it until the preparation be covered, and the top glass finally rests upon the lower one.

A quantity of fluid will yet remain outside the top glass which must be carefully taken up with the camel's hair pencil until the surface of the lower glass, around the top one, be made quite dry, when the following cement must be applied to the clean, dry glasses, to shut in the fluid, and render the preparation permanent.

Take Egyptian asphaltum and dissolve it in camphene to the consistence of a thick paste; this process is greatly facilitated by the application of moderate heat. Keep it in a well secured vessel, and label it. Then take *japanner's gold size*, which may be obtained at the varnish makers, but generally it is too thin, because new. Inspissate it by the continued application of heat until it acquire the consistence of molasses, then with a muller, upon a marble slab, grind up with the gold-size as much lamp-black as you can, until you have formed a *very stiff paste;* this should also be well secured and labelled. The properties of these ingredients are as follows:

Asphaltum is hard and brittle.

Gold-size is highly tough, and elastic, and retains these properties for many years. By combining elements respectively *too hard*, and *too* soft, the one is made to counteract the objectionable properties of the other, and the lamp-black not only assists to give good consistence to the whole, but is desirable from its indestructibility.

Japanner's gold-size is composed of boiled linseed oil, dry red lead, litharge, copperas, gum animi, and turpentine.

To use the cement, take nearly equal parts of each of the above materials, taking care that the gold-size composition should rather preponderate over the asphaltum, than the contrary; mix them intimately on a slab with a small palette knife; if too thick to work well, add a few drops of camphene, *but beware of making it too thin.* Apply the cement, thus made, with camel's hair pencil to the outer margin of the top glass; do not use too much for the first coat, but rather by successive layers, applied at different periods, fill with cement the space between the lower and upper glasses of the preparation, until a good solid layer be formed, when the process is complete. It is, however, most important *to isolate the several layers of the "black" cement,* for the turpentine contained in a newly applied coating will act upon, and partially dissolve, the old and dry layer; in this case, the upper surface being exposed to the atmosphere will speedily *dry* and *contract,* and acting upon the softened cement below the surface, will drive it between the glasses, and spoil the preparation.

Either of the following compositions may be used for the purpose of separating the layers of the black cement.

Gum arabic, ... 3 drams.
Sugar . . . . . . 1 do.
Corrosive sublimate, ... 1 grain.
Water, sufficient to make a thick mucilage.

Marine glue, dissolved in an excess of white-wood naphtha, to form a thin solution of the glue. This, which is by far the best application for the purpose, dries nearly as rapidly as it can be used. .

Having devoted upwards of thirty years of my life to the dissection of small animals by the aid of the microscope, and in the preparation of the elementary tissues of all animals, from man downwards, and being desirous of preserving and making permanent the results of my (frequently) very tedious labors, my wants, in this respect, were necessarily peculiar. The ordinary form of vessel, then, (and now,) in common use—a bottle; was altogether unsuited to my especial necessity; I could not place a *bottle* under the microscope for the examination of its contents, nor see the preparations without the microscope, the aberration, resulting from the figure of the bottle, precluding the possibility of defining with precision, the preparations contained within. Thus, the work I had been able to accomplish by suitable optical assistance could not be rendered apparent to my friends, by the use of a microscope; and whether it were an exposition of the nervous system, or other organic structure of an insect, or a minutely injected tissue of a frog, or a man, they were alike inaccessible to unassisted vision; moreover, to increase my difficulties they required to be kept as *wet* preparations. Having been in the constant habit of dissecting under water, in tin pans of various forms and sizes, and always covering these pans with a plate of glass to keep out dust, &c., when they contained unfinished dissections, or an animal simply prepared for dissection, I was struck with the beautiful appearance of an insect, or other entire animal, lying as naturally as possible, with all its full proportions displayed, retaining its characters in their utmost integrity, and so arranged as to be easy of access to the most superficial observer. To my vision, there could not be a more charming sight, than a finished dissection of the nervous system in situ of any insect, especially of the Blatta Americana—one of which I dissected at ten years of age—while lying in the pan in which the dissection had been performed; and sorely have I grieved at the sadly changed appearance of the same insect, at the instant I placed it in a bottle containing alcoholic fluid ostensibly *to preserve* it, but actually to complete its disfigurement. Neither could I suspend a delicate preparation in a bottle, in such a manner as to insure its safety. With a quantity of air always contained in the bottle, *the fluid* is put in motion by the act of taking up the vessel to examine its contents, and the particles of fluid beating against a delicate tissue will inevitably in time break or displace the structure that had cost the patient labor of many tedious hours to dissect and display. Thus, by my own act, not unfrequently, and by the carelessness of others, I was continually losing my preparations; and this determined me to attempt a form of vessel that should agree, as far as possible in all general particulars, with the pans, in which, I used then, and still continue, to dissect. Believing *glass* to be the very best material for my purpose, I consulted several operative glass-grinders on the subject; who all declared the work I required could not be done, and that if it could be accomplished, the cost would prove prohibitory. Not to be diverted from my purpose, nor discouraged by the statements of the glass-grinders, I determined to try and work out my plans with my own hands, although I had not received education in any branch of mechanics. Moreover, in connection with my project as a whole, I required a good cement for the glass vessels, and some other preserving fluid than alcohol. These subjects occupied me more or less for twenty years, during which time the failures were frequently quite disheartening, chiefly as re-garded the *mechanical* part. On one occasion, I possessed about three dozen of glass vessels, each full of fluid, hermetically sealed, and containing a minute dissection, which had remained perma-nent for a period of two years. A gas microscope had just been invented, and was then on exhibition in Bond street, London. In an evil hour I submitted my preparations to this instrument; the intense heat of the gases melted my cement, and all my treasured dissections were destroyed before my face—this occurred about eighteen years ago. In the years 1839–40 and 41, I worked most perseveringly at my glass cells, and vessels, with a view, either to complete the plan, or to give it up: at the latter end of '41 I possessed a large collection of preparations all of them contained in vessels similar to those I now use and intend to describe. I submitted them to the inspection of the Society of Arts who, having invited the assistance of a large number of eminent men, awarded me their large gold medal " for his method of putting up anatomical preparations." The medal was awarded in No-vember, '41, and presented on the distribution day in '42.* I have felt it necessary in my own justification, to give this history of a plan of mounting zoological or anatomical preparations, now in very extensive use, as I observe the method is recommended and explained in a recent publication without giving me the credit of originating and perfecting it.†

---

* The preparations here alluded to were subsequently purchased from me for £500 sterling, or $2500, by private subscription, headed by H. R. H. Prince Albert, and presented by the subscribers to the Hunterian Collection, in the Royal College of Sur-geons, where they now remain.

They were also rewarded by the late Sir Robert Peel, at that time First Lord of the Treasury, who presented me with a check, on the Royal bounty fund, for £150—$750.

† Since the above was written, a second addition has been published of the book alluded to, and the author, Mr. J. T. Quekett, has therein acknowledged my claim as the sole inventor of the plan.

There are many objects for the microscope, of great zoological or physiological interest, which possess more substance than will allow of their being treated in the way already described, although their characters can be preserved only as *wet* preparations; for all such, a *cell*, or a glass box, must now be prepared, and the following is the way to proceed.

Firstly, accurately measure the length, breadth, and substance of the preparation to be mounted; select a piece of flat glass of substance agreeing as nearly as possible with the thickness of the preparation and with a glazier's diamond cut off two pieces from one-eighth to three-sixteenths of an inch wide, and of equal length; these are to form the sides of the cell; the ends must be of the same width but not so long. Although the cell should *fit* the preparation in regard to *depth* or thickness, a good space should always be allowed around the sides and ends, for example: I desire to make a cell for a preparation measuring one inch long, and five-eighths wide, I should make the cell one and a half inch long, and one inch wide, *inside* measure; when finished the preparation looks better, is more accessible to the microscope because the sides of the vessel are not in the way, and, what is most important, *there is more room for preserving fluid*, than if the vessel be contracted to the actual size or thereabouts of its contents. The *depth* should be exact for two reasons: one, that thereby the object is retained in the center of the cell, being lightly pressed upon by the top, and bottom glasses; the other, that there being no greater substance of fluid between the object and the microscope than must needs be, a better definition of the object is obtained.

When glass is cut with a diamond it always leaves a rugged, uneven surface; for example, when broken off, one piece of glass will present a series of projections, which have left corresponding cavities in the piece to which it was attached; when placed together, they lock into each other and the addition of a thin layer of cement will form a perfect joint.

I avail myself of this fact in constructing cells of the kind just described, thus: fig. 1 represents a piece of glass of the exact length and breadth, *outside measure*, that the cell is required to be.

The two long pieces, or sides, are first cut, and before breaking them off they are marked with the scratch diamond so as to include the ends. As the width of the cell is not always sufficient to admit a number of lines, I first make a diagonal mark, then 1 and 2—rarely 3, which is unnecessary. I now separate the pieces, discard number 5, and take care to cement them to the bottom glass or slide, in the order in which they are marked, and to insure accuracy in this respect, keep the marked surface upward. As it is necessary to have a bottom glass before we can cement the pieces just cut and marked, I proceed to give some.

DESCRIPTION OF THE SLIDES.

My peculiar wants have necessitated slides of larger size than that proposed for general adoption by the Microscopical Society of London ; moreover, I had a collection of uniform preparations on slides of my size, long before that Society had existence. The slide I chiefly use measures when cut $3\frac{3}{4}$ inches, by $1\frac{5}{8}$ths : the glass should be the " patent British plate," before referred to, which being ground and polished on both sides is generally very flat : its substance varies from less than $\frac{1}{16}$th to $\frac{1}{8}$th of an inch.

Cutting Board.—To cut the slide expeditiously and uniformly it is necessary to have a *cutting board*, fig. 2. It consists of a mahogany board 11 inches by $9\frac{1}{2}$, half an inch thick and recentangular in shape ; on one of its long sides, *a*, is fastened by means of pegs or screws and glue another piece of mahogany, the *guide board*, *b*, $2\frac{1}{2}$ inches wide and $\frac{1}{4}$ thick ; this must be planed so as to be true, as the front is to form a *straight edge*. By reference to the figure it will be seen that spaces have been cut out of the guide board, the use of which will presently appear. A flat rule or gauge should be made of mahogany, 11 inches long and $\frac{1}{4}$ thick, the width to be ascertained as follows : mark out in card board a patern of the slide intended to be used, apply the glazier's diamond to a line indicating one side of the pattern and accurately measure the distance between the diamond and the other side which will give the required width of the gauge. In other words, the gauge must be of the width of the pattern, less *the* " *rake,*" (or setting) of the diamond. In addition to gauges, a *square* is essential ; the most useful is of mahogany, one-fourth of an inch thick, with sides $6\frac{1}{2}$ inches long and solid, i.e., not open,

The glass intended to be cut into slides should be placed on the cutting board, and if none of its sides have a true edge a narrow slip must be cut off its entire length to form one. The straight side of the glass must now be brought against the guide board to ascertaing if either of the sides, at right angles to the cut side be perfectly square with it; if not it is only necessary to square one side : for this purpose place the side to be squared so that it project a little beyond that part of the guide board which is cut away at *c*, apply the square, and cut of a narrow slip in in a direction contrary to the former cut : thus the two sides of the glass are made true.

Keep the glass still against the guide board and removing the square, apply the *gauge;* cut the whole length of the glass and you have the width of the slides. Now turn the squared end of the glass just cut into the space at *c*, pressing it firmly against the angles of the guide board, (which must also be made quite true,) place the gauge against the guide board in its former position, cut the glass transversely, as shewn by the dotted line, and you have the length of the slide ; and in this way cut up the remainder of the slip of glass as far it will yield slides of the proper length.

In like manner the spaces *d* and *e*, in the guide board, give the length of other slides, the width of which has been cut previously with other gauges adapted to the purpose. By this arrangement of the cutting board one gauge is alone required to cut the width and length of a slide of any given dimensions. From the forgoing description it will be obvious that the gauges must be first made, the length of the spaces in the guide board determined by their assistance, and they must be cut in it before it be affixed to the cutting board.

Grinding the Glass.—Unless the slides are to be covered with paper, the sharp, rough edges left by the diamond cut should be removed by *grinding the glass.* This can be accomplished on a perfectly flat stone of sharp grit with water; the process is greatly facilitated by the addition of emery, but a better tool, in my experience, is a plate of *soft pewter*, or the emery plate.

My pewter plate was formed in a mould made for casting the

plates on which to engrave music; its outside measure, therefore, corresponds to the size of a printed page of music, but it is ¾ of an inch thick, and weighs 14lbs. It is important that the surfaces be made quite flat, and every care should be taken to keep them so. *Soft* pewter is desirable because it contains a much greater quantity of lead than the hard, in which tin preponderates. The metal is used only as the vehicle of the cutting material, which is emery. The latter, in time, becomes thoroughly impacted in the metal, so that it will cut with the assistance of water alone, and the wear of the plate is too trifling to be estimated. When in use it should always be charged well with " superfine" emery, and water; coarser tears the glass.

In the year 1351, during a long residence in Albany, N.Y., I was enabled, with the kind assistance of my esteemed friend John E. Gavit, Esq., Bank Note Engraver of that City, to carry out a plan that had long occupied my mind in relation to forming a less weighty, and more efficient tool for grinding glass.

Constantly travelling from city to city, the *weight* of my pewter plate, together with several pounds of Emery, was a very serious task upon me, whilst the want of a fixed residence prevented me from instituting any experiments whereby I might be relieved from the incumbrance alluded to. My desire was to convert emery, by the addition of another substance, into a hard, solid, compact cake of any required dimensions, and for this purpose I believed shell-lac to be the best material. My friend caught the idea and proffered the assistance of himself and his work-shops for the purpose of seeing what could be done. Our first experiment was successful, but clearly indicating that great improvements could yet be made. We used the ingredients respectively in various proportions; submitted the plates to different degrees of pressure, and lastly, we tried emery of different degrees of fineness. Without recording our comparative failures, it is enough to say that plates composed of emery, nearly 16lbs; shell-lac, somewhat less than 2lbs; subjected to a pressure of 5 tons, have answered the best. We have used in these plates with the greatest success, Flour Emery, number O, and Superfine.

The latter cuts very fast. Of course, the emery and shell-lac can only be brought into contact by means of *heat*, and great care is necessary in melting the shell-lac, for, if the temperature be too high, or too suddenly applied, the shell-lac becomes like a mass of liver (decomposed), and you can do nothing with it.

Neither is it the easiest thing imaginable to knead so small a quantity of shell-lac with the large quantity of emery already stated. Success, however, depends upon this operation being well performed.

Subjected to *moderate* pressure, the plate will cut glass *incredibly fast*, but at the expense of the plate which will wear nearly through in a few hours.

The plates made under a pressure of 5 tons (in my occupation) have been used constantly and severely for 14 months without any sensible diminution. My desire to submit these plates to the severe test of time and use, induced me in this, as on many previous occasions to delay publishing any account of them, notwithstanding I once more laid myself open to the piracies of unprincipled and unscrupulous men.

These plates are round, some of mine as much as 10 inches in diamater, and from $\frac{5}{16}$ths to $\frac{3}{8}$ths thick. Although the plates were pressed between *two level metallic surfaces*, they yet require grinding to make them true; this is easily accomplished by means of superfine emery and plenty of water, and as in the course of time and use this operation requires to be repeated, it is necessary to have two such plates, and as each plate possesses' *two* surfaces, it is easy to obtain truth by grinding the sides interchangeably.

To use these plates for grinding, it is only necessary to keep the surfaces well wetted with water.

Unlike the pewter plate, the emery plate can be advantageously employed for grinding sections of bone, teeth, spines of echini, the selerogenous tissues of plants or fossils: in the former instrument the loose, sharp cutting emery becomes impacted in the tissues *and never can be removed*, but in the latter the emery is too tightly held by the shell-lac and cannot get into any tissue. The only sensible wear is, not of the *emery*, but in the shell-lac; and thus, occasionally, the plate will cease to cut, and the surface will be covered with a gummy something which keeps the glass or other material from actual contact with the emery—this is shell-lac.

If you now wash the surface of the plate evenly with alcohol, or Liquor Potassæ which is better, the shell-lac will be dissolved, and this should be well washed off with a copious stream of water—the well cleaned teeth of the emery will now cut sharper than ever.

When my friend had acquired, what the Yankees call " the hang of it " he made a batch of these plates (some 50 or 60) believing them to be important in many mechanical operations no less than to supply his own wants; some of these he intended to sell, and for all that I know to the contrary, they may yet be procured from him by those persons who have not the tools for making them, but would like to possess such appliances.

Hold the glass slide to be ground at an angle of about 45 °, that *the outer line of the edge* may alone touch the plate of metal: grind by a quick, light, circular motion—to and from, round the corners—until the line be straight and beveled; change the position of the glass to grind the *opposite* outer line in the same manner; now hold the glass vertically, and make the edge smooth. By beveling the outsides of the edge of glass in the first instance they are saved from breaking, which is inevitable without this precaution; it is true that beveling can be done at any time, but it is not easy to grind out the deep irregular holes caused by splitting the edge. In this way, the four sides of the slide are to be ground.

To keep the pewter plate, or emery plate flat, grinding should invariably be conducted all over its surface; but as this is somewhat difficult with small pieces of glass on a large surface of metal, I devote one side of my plate for slides alone, and reserve the other for purposes where the utmost flatness is necessary. Its flatness, however, should be frequently tested with a straight edge, and if elevations appear, they should be reduced by grinding them down. Optical glass grinders and other mechanics, who require a plane grinding surface, have three similar tools; when one of them becomes untrue by use, it is ground with one of the others,

until they present a like surface, neither of them true. Tool No.
1 being now ground with tool No. 3, the inequalities left by No.
2 are obliterated, and a flat surface is the result. As it would be
particularly inconvenient for me to carry with me three plates
each weighing 14 lbs. for the sake of keeping one of them true,
I resort to another, but equally efficient plan: I take a piece of
plate glass of the same length as the pewter plate, the width not
being very material, with plenty of emery and water I grind the
metal all over its surface with the *flat* side of the glass until they
present a corresponding surface; if the metal be not sufficiently
flat, I turn the glass and grind the other side: by this process the
flatness of the metal may be insured; with the surfaces of the
shell-lac and emery plates the correction, as before described, is
very simple.

To abbreviate the time of edging the slides, it is expedient
to hold one in each hand and grind them simultaneously; and
although this may be somewhat difficult at first, a little practice
will give all the facility and tact necessary for thus grinding *two*
glasses in the time of one.

Cement for the Cells.—The slide being ready, the cell is to be
cemented to it, and for this purpose a good, and water-proof cement is necessary. Canada balsam is too brittle; gum mastic is
equally brittle and difficult to use, and I could not for some years
find anything equal in toughness and durability to my own composition—gold size and lamp black—and I have now in my possession cells containing wet preparations cemented with it 14
years ago, every portion of which is perfectly sound. It is, however, in every respect, vastly inferior to the marine glue already
alluded to. In the year 1842 my attention was directed to this
composition by the newspaper accounts of experiments made with
it at the Royal dockyards at Woolwich.

I consulted the patentee, Mr. Jeffery, and desired to know if
it could be applied as a cement to glass; of this he knew nothing, and gave me some to try, and general directions how to use
it. It failed; and for some months continued to fail, until the
inventor made some specially for my use at the College of Surgeons, with which I had the most complete success. As made
for general use, the marine glue consists of different degrees of

hardness, distinguished by numbers, from one, downwards; the particular composition made for me agreed nearly with the ordinary " No. 4," but as in addition to caoutchouc and shell-lac— the staple ingredients of the marine glue—this contained another and most important material, as applied to glass, it was agreed to call it " No. 4, G. K. ;" subsequently the same valuable in-gredient enters into the composition of every form of marine glue, so that " No. 4 " is now a sufficient description of it.

Another and very beautiful preparation of the marine glue has been made in the United States, suggested by Dr. P. B. God-dard of Philadelphia.

It consists of caoutchouc dissolved in chloroform by the ap-plication of gentle heat to the consistence of a thick mucilage-nous paste ; then add clean, carefully selected tears of gum mas-tic, until the composition becomes sufficiently liquified to use with a brush, when it should be filtered to free it from the dirt always combined with the gums in question. The gum mastic not only readily dissolves in chloroform, but it is a somewhat cu-rious fact that it should reduce the thick solution of India rubber to the condition of a transparent, lympid fluid ; it must not be made too thin however, for when dry it will be brittle from the excess of mastic. This is a very elegant cement; it can be used with or without heat, and when dry it possesses the great advantage of being perfectly colorless and transparent: I have not employed it for vessels of much size, but simply for shallow cells.* The patent marine glue requires heat, and I have already described one mode of melting it; the following is the way *to cement the cells.*

Aparatus used in cementing the Cells.—I employ for this pur-pose an aparatus that I made many years ago for mounting prep-arations in Canada balsam. It forms an important part of the contents of my " manipulating box," and it is one of the things pirated by the author of the modern work indicated.

A plate of wrought iron $6\frac{3}{8}$ths by $2\frac{3}{8}$ths and $\frac{1}{8}$th thick, ground

---

* Since writing the above, I find that the preparations for which I used it 12 months before have not stood, I cannot, therefore, recommend it.

on its upper surface,)fig. 3 *a* is supported by four legs of brass wire (*d*) $\frac{3}{16}$ths diamater, and 3 inches long in the clear;* they screw into holes at the corners of the iron plate, and their free ends are placed in sockets in a mahogany board (*b*) the size of the iron plate, and $\frac{1}{4}$ thick. When in use, the plate becomes so hot that it cannot be touched with the hand, and the legs by conducting the heat, mark the table; to render the entire aparatus more convenient, I found it better to add the mahogany board; the holes for the legs are defended with brass plates, and they fit tightly, so that the whole can be moved bodily out of the operator's way. The spirit lamp (*c*) is $1\frac{1}{4}$ inch square and $2\frac{1}{4}$ high to the top of the brass wick holder—exclusive of the ground glass cap. Every part of the glass that is to be coated with the marine glue should firstly be lightly painted with the fluid solution of it before described. Thus prepared, the slide and the four pieces of the cell should be placed on the iron plate, and the heat of the lamp applied beneath.

The position of the lamp should be frequently changed, to impart an equal temperature to the iron plate, for if there be too great an accumulation of heat at any one point, the glass will instantly break; should the plate become unnecessarily hot, lower the wick, or remove the lamp for a short time.

The solid glue may be cut into long thin slips with a knife or scissors, and applied to the painted surface of the slide and pieces of the cell, until the glass be hot enough to melt it, when it should be distributed evenly over the glass by means of another piece of glue held in a pair of short, strong forceps. Then search for, and remove, particles of grit and dirt which are contained more or less in the glue—they are best seen by removing the glass from the iron plate and placing it on a piece of clean, dry, white paper; they can be easily removed by the point of a knife, or a piece of the solid glue. Extraneous particles are frequently broken into fragments between the glasses by the pressure necessary to form a joint, but they should always be removed, as they act mechanically as a wedge, and preclude the possibility of a permanent joint.

---

* The height of the spirit lamp must determine the *length* of the legs.

At a certain temperature the glue will bubble and boil, at which point it should be removed from further contact with heat ; otherwise it will be decomposed, and all its characteristics destroyed.*

For neatness and uniformity, the cells should be placed in the centre of the slides, and to accomplish this it is best to mark the outline of the slide on paper or card-board with a pen, and then draw a cross, the centre of which is the centre of the slide, its limbs extending the whole length of the long and the short diameter of the figure.

The glass being hot, and the glued surfaces freed from dirt, the several pieces of the cell are to be turned quickly over with a pair of forceps, and placed upon the slide in the relative position they should occupy.

The slide should now be put on the card-board figure, each piece of the cell should be pressed down to the slide with two pieces of wood, and rubbed to and fro to express the excess of glue, and make as near approach to contact with the lower glass as is compatible with the thinnest layer of glue. The four pieces of the cell having been cemented to the slide and to each other, its position can be readily adjusted to the centre, by the aid of the cross figured on the card. Should the glass become a little too cool and the glue set, replace it on the iron plate and complete the adjustment.

Before the glass and the glue become quite cold and hard, it is desirable to remove the superfluous glue which holds most pertinaceously when cold : the best form of instrument for this purpose is the lozenge-shaped tool used by engravers, keeping the point close to the sides of the joint, or a knife-point may be used, taking care not to scratch the glass. As a rule, it must be borne in mind that, whenever a cell consists of more than one piece of glass, it should be ground flat on the pewter or emery plate, after being glued to the slide before it is fit to be trusted : the slightest inequality, either in the substance of the glass at

---

* This is the peculiar decomposition of the shell-lac before described.

one end, or in the layer of the marine glue, will prevent the possibility of making a good joint hereafter with the top glass or cover.

To clean the glass perfectly, I use a small piece of cotton wool gathered into a knot, held by a pair of strong steel forceps, and a drop or two of liquor potassæ, or a saturated solution of caustic potash, which softens the marine glue and admits of its removal. Care must be taken not to allow the potash to remain in contact with the joints, as it decomposes the glue, and will render the joints unsound. The glass should be well rinsed in a large quantity of clean water, to remove the potash.

A top glass or cover must now be cut for the cell, and this should be somewhat smaller than the outer diameter of the cell on all sides, to allow room for the cement. The edges of the cover, and surface of the cell, should be painted with the naphtha solution of marine glue; and the cell will then be ready for the reception of the preserving fluid, and the preparation. It is best to fill the cell over some other vessel to catch the excess of fluid that is sure to run over the sides; a small shallow dish or saucer will answer this purpose; and if the cell be supported upon a level something placed in the dish, the better, as the operator will have his hands at liberty.

Having filled the cell with fluid, take a short but strong camel's (or badger's) hair pencil, and rub the fluid into the corners, along the sides of the cell, and even the bottom glass, for this reason: in pouring the fluid into the cell, it remains separated from the glass in every direction by a filmy layer of atmospheric air, which can only be removed, and the fluid and glass brought in contact mechanically, or by the thin gum-water, or saliva, formerly referred to. If a vessel be sealed down without attending to this precaution, the air will de liberated by degrees and form a great number of minute bubbles, glistening in rows upon the sides, in the angles of the cell, and even upon the bottom glass:—ultimately they coalesce, and an air bubble of some size is the result. For the same reason (the displacement of air), the preparation must be placed carefully in the cell, and if it, possess cavities in the under surface, they should be pressed out if possible, while the preparation is entering the cell; and this should be managed so that one end of the preparation goes into the vessel first, and the remainder lowered gradually. A good steady stream of fluid should be poured into the cell, the prepa· ration being held down by a camel's hair pencil or forceps, until all extraneous particles be washed away, and the fluid continue bright and clear. When at rest the fluid in the cell will present a *convex surface*, bounded on all ·sides by the painting of marine glue.

Now prepare one surface of the cover, either by the tongue or brushing on the fluid as before, and holding it by a pair of for- ceps at one end of its *longest* diameter, lower the other end to the cell, and let it down gradually—the excess of fluid running be- fore—until it be in its place; then adjust it accurately; press down the cover till it touch evenly every part of the bed on which; it is to rest, remove with a brush whatever fluid may yet remain on the outer edges, and paint them *once* more with the naphtha solution, including this time the top glass : apply the black ce- ment, and the preparation is finished. Should another layer of black cement be required, allow the first to become quite dry, and isolate it, as before directed, with the napththa solution; successive layers of the black cement must always be thus separated.

Drilling or cutting circular holes in glass for cells.—A more ele- gant mode of constructing a cell, is by drilling a circular hole through a piece of glass (fig. 4) ; but when I first attempted this plan, (in the years 1839–40,) the cost was prohibitory. At last I employed at the same time, three workmen in London to ascer- tain the lowest rate of cost at which holes of all sizes could be drilled in glass, in any quantity not less than one gross. Neither of these men employed the same means ; one of them, a German, cut most beautiful cells, perfectly square inside, but he could not do them for less than 1s. 6d. or 36 cents each.

Another made very indifferent cells at 1s. or 24 cents each ; and the third made excellent work at 6d. or 12 cents each. Sub- sequently, another man undertook to do them equally well for half that sum, and ultimately I procured them at the same price, excellently cut, from Mr. Dennis of 1 Charles street, St. John's Street Road, London. The following is the plan of proceeding : procure a copper tube (or drill, as it is called) of the diameter you desire your cell to be : I have long since discontinued cells of *all* sizes, and chiefly use one of 1¾ths diameter, cut out of a square of glass 1½ inch *full*, outside measure.

With my large slides such a cell enables me to preserve great uniformity in my preparations, affords abundant space for the transmission of light around the object, holds a sufficient quantity of preserving fluid, and the squares can be cut with the same guage used for the slides themselves. The length of the drill may be from 1 inch to 1½ long, and made to run true in a lathe. The squares of glass being all of the same size, I cement a number of them together with the marine glue, so as to form a pile of from one inch to two inches high.

Where a *lathe* is used, it is important to face the pile of squares with something that has been already perforated with a hole the size of the drill to enable the latter to enter at once upon its work, and prevent the scratching (and spoiling) the first cell. For this purpose, *brass* perfectly flat, can be used ; but a better thing is a square of *plate glass*, one-fourth of an inch thick, already perforated by the same drill, and it should be kept for this purpose alone.

The copper drill is to be charged with fine cutting sand and water, and the block, or pile of glass squares applied to it, and gradually pressed up by the tail spindle of the lathe, while the drill should revolve at a *moderate*, but not a *rapid* rate. When a number of cells are drilled, they can be easily separated from the block by placing the outer cell downwards on the iron plate and applying the spirit lamp : they can be removed one after the other with great rapidity, untill only *undrilled* glasses remain, and to these other squares may be added if necessary. To make an oval cell, two round holes (fig. 5, *a*, *b*,) must be drilled so as to intersect each other ; their proximity to be determined by the *length* of the oval required. The pieces that remain on each side, *c*, *d*, can be cut off with the diamond if the glass do not exceed one-eighth of an inch thick, otherwise a disc of copper, the diameter of a ten cent piece must be applied to the lathe, charged with, sand and water on the edge, and it will speedily make the sides of the cell level.

There is another excellent method of cutting either round or oval cells of any size, *provided the glass do not exceed one-eighth inch in thickness,* for which I am indebted to Sir Charles Babbage, the inventor of the celebrated calculating machine.   Mount a glazier's diamond to cut a circle ; this can be done in a variety of ways—I have mounted my diamond as shown in fig. 6. *a* represents a square bar of iron, 8 inches long, with a male screw at the lower end to fit a plate of iron (*i*) tapped to receive it, *b, b,* two arms 4½ inches long, clamped to the upright bar by thumb screws, the other extremity drilled and ground to receive *c,* which is a spindle, to the lower end of which is rivetted a screwed rod *d,* 4 inches long from the centre.   *e* is a box to receive the glazier's diamond when removed from the handle, and kept in its place by a tightening screw ; continuous with this box is a square nut, *f,* perforated with a hole large enough to allow it to swing freely on the screwed arm.   *g, g,* are square screwed nuts, one on each side of the diamond box.

In adjusting the diamond to cut a disc, say three inches diamater, move it along the screwed arm until the point be coincident with 3 inches as marked upon the scale (*l*) which has before been drawn upon the chamois leather which covers the board K ; then bring the nuts close to either side of the diamond box, adjust it to its cutting angle, and then by means of a wrench in each hand *tighten* the nuts simultaneously.   The glass to be cut may now be placed upon the board ; remove the pin *h,* and lower the spindle (*c*) till the diamond touch the glass : then holding the screwed arm by one hand, turn it steadily round and it will describe a circle of the size to which the diamond has been previously adjusted.

As the spindle has been ground to fit the two collars through which it works, the motion is smooth and steady.   Such a machine would be improved by casting the upright bar and the two arms, *b, b,* in one piece ; the height need not exceed six inches. Having cut a circle on a piece of glass, if the *disc* be wanted, cut the glass in three or four places *from the circular cut to the outer edge,* and carefully break off the pieces; but if a *cell* be wanted, the *disc must be removed* without injury to the remainder of the glass, which is to form the walls of the required cell.

The cut, already made, gives the exact dimensions of the aperture required; now alter the position of the diamond on the screwed arm and cut a circle *within* the first, adjust again and cut another circle within the last, and so proceed cutting circle within circle as long as the diamond can be adjusted to cut, and the glass will then present a series of concentric circles.

Take a centre punch and screw it point upwards in a bench vice; place the centre of the *innermost circle* on the point of the punch, and get an assistant to hold the glass while the operator takes another centre punch and placing its point *upon* the glass immediately over the point of the lower punch strike the upper punch lightly with a hammer, *not to break,* but to *pound* the glass lying between the two punches. Presently a small hole will be made; now bring the broken edge of the glass upon the lower punch continuing the pounding motion until the hole be sufficiently enlarged to admit of using the "*plane*" of the small and light hammer with which the punch has been struck. At this stage of the process, the use of the upper punch should be discontinued, and the operator holding the glass himself, *keeping an edge of the hole always supported on the lower punch* while he lightly taps it with the plane of the hammer, not attempting to remove the *circles* as cut, but rather tracing the hole from the *centre to the circumference,* (like making a cross in the glass,) and if it have been *cut,* not *scratched,* large pieces will fall out as soon as they have room enough, and the entire operation be finished in less time than it takes to describe it.

In like manner, an oval cell can be made as easily as a round one. The glass should not be cut into shape to form the *outer* dimensions of the cell, until the central hole be made, as it is likely to break. Upon this plan a hole of any size can easily be cut in a plate of glass of any dimensions. Sir Charles Babbage told me that he once communicated this plan to a glazier, who employed it most extensively in punching holes in squares

of glass to form the bottom plates of street gas lamps, for the transmission of the gas pipe.

I have already remarked, that the above plan of cell-making
is limited to glass one-eighth of an inch thick; my wants frequently require cells full as deep again; I could cement two or
more shallow ones together, and thus build up any required
depth, but they look heavy, and I prefer therefore to cut them out
of plate glass of the proper thickness. When in London, I could
obtain the services of Mr. Dennis to cut anything that I required,
at any time; but in this country, at this moment, I am altogether
thrown upon my own resources. To meet my wants I have contrived a small, portable, and most efficient apparatus, by means
of which any lad can cut cells as well as I can, and with this
machine my Son has cut for me the best cells I have ever had.

It consists of *a, a,* (fig. 7, A,) an iron support with three arms
and a square plate at the lower end of it, cast in one piece. *b,* a
vertical bevelled wheel working *c,* a horizontal beveled wheel
by means of the crank *d,* the latter wheel, having for its axis a
spindle *e,* the lower end of which screws into the brass mount
of the copper drill, *f,* whilst its other end passes through a collar
in the upper arm of the iron support and is regulated in its action
by the wooden lever *g.*

Attached to the under surface of the wooden lever is a strong
steel spring, about one inch wide, the profile of which is shown
at B, fig. 7. *m* is the spring, to be screwed to the lever by the
flat extremities. In the centre of the curved portion there is a
slit through which the upper part of the spindle *n,* previously
reduced for that purpose, passes, and in which it can freely play;
it is kept in its place by the button *o.*

The square plate *i,* (A and C,) is screwed down to the board *j,*
by four nut-headed screws. *h, h,* are two thick pieces of wood
screwed on to the bottom board *j,* their inner edges being under
cut to form a bevelled groove in which the two pieces of wood
marked *k,* being beveled to the same angle, may freely move.

In the centre of the pieces marked *k* is a slit, through which
passes a nut-headed screw to connect them with the lower board

and to admit of their adjustment, their inner extremities are cut to form half a square and are intended to receive the block of glass placed diagonally, to be drilled by the machine. The block of glass, *l*, should be placed exactly in the centre, and it can easily be secured in its position by clamping the side pieces of wood by means of the nut-headed screws and collars.

With this machine I employ superfine emery and water. It cuts best by a *dragging* motion; pulling the crank half round with one hand whilst the lever is kept down with the other; and then lifting up the lever and allowing *the crank to go the other half round without grinding.* By alternately lifting up the lever and pressing it down, the emery works into the cut; whereas if the lever be kept steadily down, either by a weight, or by the hand, and the crank turned constantly round, the drill will be cut away much faster than the glass.

The fixed position of the horizontal beveled wheel, *c*, would seem to preclude the possibility of elevating the spindle, *e*, the required height.

To obviate this difficulty, a notch is made in the wheel *c*, into which a square steel plug $1\frac{1}{2}$ inch long is driven, which works freely in a corresponding slab made in the spindel, *e*.

The same directions apply to cementing the round and oval cells to the slides as those already given; and when finished they appear like fig. 8, where *a* represents the slide, *b* the cell cemented to it, and *c* the *well* formed for the reception of the preparation and the fluid.

Cells cut out of the *very thin glass*, that which is usually employed for covers rarely answer, *for want of flatness* in the glass itself; and yet, a great number of very beautiful and valuable, microscopical preparations, of the animal and vegetable kingdoms can only be preserved *in fluid*, and by the introduction of some medium to defend them from pressure between an upper and lower plate of glass. For this purpose I have long employed the marine glue, as the material from which to construct *very shallow cells.* Subsequently, the same substance has been employed by others for a like purpose, as Vide Quekett's Treatise

on the microscope; but the modus operandi, as therein described, differs so essentially from my plan that I think it expedient to
give a description of it.

For neatness sake it is desirable that the cell, whether round or
oval, should be placed in the *centre* of the slide, and to ensure accuracy in this respect together with rapidity of action I made a
tool described in the accompanying figure, 9.

a Is a flat board of the substance represented in the figure;
b b b, are three pieces of wood raised upon *a*, and so placed that
a space is left, *c*, from front to back; this is intended to fit the
bottom glass, on which a cell is to be made, and should fit the
short diameter of the glass so well that it can only just pass in and
out; in other words, room to admit of lateral motion is objectionable. The space is not intended to be as long as the greater
diameter of the glass. *d*, Represents a thinner piece of wood
fastened to the sides of the frame *b b*, in the centre of which is a
round hole—the size of this hole can only be regulated by the
width of the glass. One size slide that I have long used is less
than that recommended by the Microscopical Society; and I
have drawn the figure to exact dimensions of the apparatus, it is
intended to represent. The round hole is intended to receive and
form a guide for a round copper, brass, or tin tube—copper
being the best. The exact position of the perforated cross piece
of wood can only be ascertained (as will soon appear) from
actual experiment.

Having determined the size of the slip of glass upon which a
cell of marine glue is to be formed, it is necessary to determine
the diameter of the circle which is to form the *interior* margin of
the cell.

Procure a tube of copper, brass, or tin, about three inches
long, the *outside* diameter of which corresponds with the *internal*
margin above described. Especial care should be taken to
have a sufficient space outside the circle and the sides of the glass
slide to form a good support for the top glass, and for the black
cement to secure it.

The hole in the cross piece *e*, must allow the tube to work easily through it, and the cross piece so fitted to the frame, that when the glass slide is placed in the space *c*, the tube placed in the hole in the cross piece will descend upon the *exact centre* of the slide, equi-distant from end to end, equi-distant from side to side. The accurate adjustment of the cross piece is somewhat troublesome ; for *circular* cells, it is not very important ; but for oval cells it becomes a necessity.

This apparatus being ready, place the glass slide on the iron plate and apply the spirit lamp ; put some marine glue on the glass and as it melts distribute it evenly over the glass to an extent *beyond the proposed limits of the cell*; the *quantity* of the glue must depend upon the depth of cell required. If it be wanted *very shallow*, continue the application of heat to procure the necessary hardness of the glue, but in all cases the glue should be made tolerably hard by inspissation. Remove the glass slide from the iron plate to space *c*, in the wooden frame, dip the end of the metal tube in water, pass it through the guide aperture in the cross piece, press it firmly upon the glued surface of the glass slide, turn it half round and remove it—a circle will be cut in the hot glue on the glass; the interior of which can be (now) easily removed, the water from the tube assisting.

It is easy to make an *oval* cell of any dimensions in the *long* diameter commensurate with the size of the apparatus, in this way : cut some pieces of glass the exact width of the space *c*, ¼th, ¼th, ⅜ths, &c., wide ; place one of these in the frame close up to *f*, now put the glass slide in its place, resting against, not the wood *f*, but the narrow glass placed there ; make the round hole in the hot marine glue with this punch, instantly *turn* the slide end for end, and punch again, remove it, and with a knife connect the *axes* of the two circles, clean off the glue from the interior, and the oval is made. If the aperture in the cross pieces be other than exact, the oval will be *diagonal* in respect to the long diameter of your slide.

Now grind the cell upon the emery plate to the required substance—it can be made beautifully flat,—and then by means of a square and knife form the outer lines of the square in which your round hole is punched, or the ends of your oval cell, as the case may be : my *small* slides are so narrow that the space beyond the circle in the smaller diameter is only enough to give a required margin for the cover, and cement.

A little piece of cotton wool, dipped in liq : potassæ, held in a pair of forceps, and applied to the interior of the cell, will soften the glue, and it can then be easily removed with a scalpel, small chisel (⅜th diameter), or lozenge shaped engravers' tool. When finished, the cell is really a beautiful one ; I have never had a preparation in this form of cell *fail.*

In a former publication devoted to a description of my preserving fluids and glass cells, my silence with regard to one particular form of cell, also of my invention, was misconstrued by a gentleman who has, it appears, adopted my cast-off. I allude to a cell made by cutting off a slice of a glass tube.

In the year 1841 being in Edinburgh, I employed the late Mr. Sanderson, Lapidary of the Pleasance, to make sections of glass tubes for my use, but, as he could not make two sides alike or either of them true, they failed. Sections of a tube can only be made true by a compound motion of this kind, i. e., they must not only be ground with a circular motion on a flat surface, but revolve on their own axis simultaneously.

If such a disc be firmly held by the thumb and finger and submitted to the grinding process already described, the *pressure being unequal,* it will cut quicker beneath the finger and thumb than elsewhere, and still more beneath the thumb than the finger : change its position and you have the like result, so that *holes* or *hollows* must be formed unless the disc can be made to revolve *constantly and uniformly,* subject to the same pressure.

With such a surface, it is hopeless to expect to obtain contact with flat glass, and marine glue,

Apparently you have a joint : but if the preparation be subject to the slightest jar at any time, off comes the slice of tube cell and the preparation is lost. A friend of mine, resident at Albany, being in New York city, purchased 12 injected preparations just arrived from London. Six of these were mounted in the section of tube cell, the remainder in cells drilled out of flat glass—a round hole in the small square plate. On his arrival at home, his children anxious to see all that had arrived from New York, clutched at the table cover on which the rarities were displayed, down went the 12 slides, and when picked up, the six *drilled* holes in the square plates of glass were uninjured, the other six had separated and the *costly* preparations were entirely lost ; nothing would induce that man to purchase preparations mounted in cells of that form again. Where it necessary, I could give a great number of like illustrations; but I think it must be obvious, that the four corners of a square glass with a round hole in it must cling with great pertinacity to the lower plate, and that, if it be possible (as it really is) to cement two pieces of glass together so firmly that no mechanical force can separate them, this should give a better chance of success than a thin rim of glass.

I can only add that amidst my incessant wanderings on this side of the Atlantic, I have more than once, twice or thrice, been horrified to see a box containing upwards of 60 dozen of long cherished and much valued preparations *flung out of a waggon*, or hurled to the ground from a baggage waggon in a manner peculiar to railway travelling in the United States, and such as no one who has once seen it can ever forget, and yet, only twice out of 3 years have my preparations been broken, and on *each occasion* the ends, only, of bottom glasses were broken off close to the *outer margin of the cell*; in no one instance has a *cell come off.*

There are many preparations of entire animals no less than dissected portions of them, which can be well displayed only in vessels with flat surfaces, in contradistinction to round or oval bottles ; but, from their greater size, they cannot be contained in vessels constructed on the principle of those already described. For all such, I build up a *box* of glass, consisting of four sides, the bottom plate (or slide) and the top, or cover—six pieces in all.

These vessels are confessedly difficult to make; yet they form the most attractive and beautiful exhibitions that can be put into a museum. The trouble I have had with these upright vessels, no less than my great desire to submit them and the preserving fluids, to the only satisfactory test—time, has retarded the publication, on my part, of the several processes herein referred to.

Having settled the length, depth, and width for an upright box, the glass for the sides should be selected of sufficient substance for the bulk and weight of fluid the vessel is destined to contain; and it will frequently happen that the ends (by which I mean the two lengths of *least diameter*, calling the larger and outer portions the sides, as in the annexed figure, 10,) require to be somewhat thicker than the sides to insure sufficient surface for a joint. The glass should be cut as true and square as possible in the first instance; the two side pieces and the two end pieces should be connected together, respectively, with the marine glue, forming two pairs of glasses. First, bevel all the glasses, on the metal or emery plate, as before directed; and then proceed to make perfectly flat the extreme ends of each pair of glasses; this, the most important, is, at the same time the most difficult part of the work, and such as can be accomplished only by practice; the position of the glass in the hand must be frequently changed, for the pressure of two fingers on one side, opposed to the thumb on the other, will have a tendency to incline the glass to an angle of 45°, whilst the operator believes he is holding it perfectly upright. It frequently saves time to grind till a smooth but inclined surface extend from one outer edge of the pair of glasses to the other, and then change its position in the hand—the probability is, that there will be the like tendency to form a similar angle, although reversed, and by carefully watching and measuring, the operation may be suspended at the point where perfect flatness obtains, and just before the inclined plane can be formed in the other direction. A small brass Square will be found of considerable importance in testing the truth of the grinding, but the most severe test is that which I always resort to namely, to wet the ground surface of glass as lightly as possible and place on it a plate of plate-glass—the sides of which, for all practical purposes, are parallel : if true and flat, the plate-glass will be seen to touch every part of the ground surface and form with it a **T**. Now wipe all the glass just tested quite dry; *breathe* upon the ground surface, and quickly apply the plate-glass—if true, the moisture of the breath will be equally diffused along its surface, and the contact be so perfect that the ground surface will hang suspended for several seconds from the plate-glass. If the work endure this test, there need be no difficulty in making a permanent joint.

Again use the iron-plate, un-cement and clean the glasses, prepare the ground surfaces of the ends and the flat surfaces of the sides against which the ends are to abut, with the naphtha solution ; return all the glass to the iron-plate (if small enough to lie there at the same time) and place marine glue on the painted flat surfaces of the sides ; when melted put on the *ends*, which will form three sides of an open square, then quickly place the other side on the ends, and carefully remove it from the plate to a piece of wood, or paper—the former, provided with a straight edge (like the cutting board) is the best. While the glass remains hot enough to keep the glue soft, press together and critically adjust the glued surfaces, taking especial care that the sides coincide with the angles of the brass square ; it is most important to remove from the glue in the joints any extraneous particles of dirt. These preliminaries settled, the glass cold, and the glue hard, the operator will have four sides of a box—like a brick-maker's mould—without top or bottom ; this he may now proceed to grind upon the metal or emery plate, firstly bevelling the edges, by a circular motion—constantly turning the box in his hand to prepare it for the bottom : after this is accomplished, it must pass the ordeal of the former test next the slide or bottom plate of glass must be heated on the iron plate, (it having been previously prepared with the naphtha solution which must also be applied to the ground surface of the box ;) and then after melting the marine glue on the upper surface near the edge for the adhesion of the lower edges of the hollow box, this box is to be applied to the slide and the whole suffered to remain on the heated plate of iron long enough for the lower portion of the sides of the box to become sufficiently hot to form a joint with the slide, but without melting the joints previously made; if it can be avoided when cold, the upper surface may be ground in the same manner as the bottom, and with like care, and when finished, the vessel will appear like figure 10.

To give additional support and resistance to the joints, Mr. Dennis, suggested to me the application of triangular bars of glass, which he called " angle pieces " cemented into the corners. In my experience of them they fail, for two reasons—one, because they cannot be ground with sufficient accuracy, and the other, that in cementing them the heat is generally so great as to decompose the glue. I have substituted the following plan with more success: I pour melted glue into the corners, and make the angles of the vessel hot enough to keep the glue fluid, while I cause it to run equally from the bottom to the top of the box— this plan has not disappointed my expectation of it in any instance.

I have made several upright vessels some of them of great dimensions (fifteen inches high, six inches wide, and four inches deep) and extremely elegant in their appearance. A preparation of Physalia pelagica (Portuguese Man of War), fig 11, will give an idea of this form of vessel ; the original box is eight inches high by two inches wide, five-eighths deep from back to front: *a* represents the front side. *b b*, the end pieces, *c*, a block of pollished plate-glass half an inch thick to which the upright box is cemented, *d*, a thinner plate of glass forming with *c* a handsome pedestal and heavy support for the upright vessel.*

The joints of the pedestal, and of the box to the thick upper plate, must be made with Canada balsam or the *chloroform* preparation of marine glue for the sake of transparency ; the box must be made as before directed, with the patent marine glue. When

*The mode of grinding a box of the height here mentioned, does not in any respect differ from that which has been described. Here the end pieces are considerably elongated, and must firstly be made true in the direction of their longer axis—the top and bottom is not to be ground untill the hollow box be perfect.

large surfaces of glass are to be cemented together, the iron-plate is insufficient for the purpose and another plan must be had recourse to. I have already remarked that a red-hot soldering iron may be applied to the edges of glass with considerable impunity, and I use such in the manufacture of large upright vessels. Fig. 12 represents the several forms of such irons as I have found desirable. Numbers 1, 2, 3, and 6, are reduced one-half in size; and five is more reduced; 1 and 2 are made of iron rod ^{5} ths inch square, welded to a round iron wire which is inserted into a wooden handle; 2 only differs from 1 in having the iron wire bent as shown in the figure—they are both eleven inches long, inclusive; 3 is intended to apply the marine glue to the inner angles of the boxes and upright vessels; an end view is shown at 4. The wire of this last is differently fixed, and its length, including the wooden handle, is fifteen inches; 5 represents a much heavier tool and is designed to retain the heat for a longer time than either of the former. With a pair of such instruments, large surfaces of glass can be well and expeditiously soldered.

To be concluded in the next number.

*** The Publisher begs to inform the Subscribers of the Upper Canada Medical Journal, that the diagrams referred to in the above communication, are in the hands of the Artist, and will be forthcoming at the conclusion of the article in the next number.

Meteorological Register.

MONTHLY METEOROLOGICAL REGISTER, AT

Latitude, 43 deg. 39.4 min. N. Longitude, 79 deg. 21.5 min. W.

Magt.	Day	Barometer * Corrected.				Temperature of the air.†				Tension of Vapour.			
		6, A.M.	2, P.M.	10,P M.	MEAN.	6.A.M.	2, P.M.	10,P M	MEAN'	6.A.M.	2, P.M.	10,P.M	MEAN.
c	1	0.317	0.332	0.284	0:306	2.8	7.9	1.7	4.26	0.147	0.187	0.157	0.167
bd	2	.307	.322	.268	.289	0.1	10.4	1.3	3.84	.139	.206	.154	.167
c	3	.162	.092	.044	.053	5.1	10.7	13.8	9.93	.169	.217	.264	.215
b	4	.271	.323	.328	.307	14.5	10.5	6.5	10.68	.244	.265	.216	.237
c	5	.253	.176	....	....	13.2	10.4	...	....	.236	.244	....	....
c	6	.121	.266	.314	.239	13.3	10.7	17.2	13.83	.238	.256	.290	.256
c	7	.281	.495	.636	.478	18.6	18.3	17.1	18.21	.274	.341	.281	.296
c	8	.379	.164	.073	.193	13.2	8.1	7.5	9.78	.228	.159	.158	.179
bc	9	.151	.237	.180	.186	11.4	7.5	4.8	7.71	.189	.186	.169	.179
•	10	.059	.044	.060	.066	1.7	9.5	3.7	5.01	.135	.179	.161	.153
•	11	.170	.233	.174	.194	6.1	5.5	2.9	5.09	.160	.159	.124	.144
•	12	.071	.019	....	....	4.1	3.2	...	....	.126	.131	...,	....
cd	13	.060	.022	.162	.631	1.4	1.0	1.8	0.71	.118	.164	.108	.132
c	14	.336	.389	.318	.343	3 8	0 9	3.1	0.09	.105	.172	.137	.125
b	15	.324	+429	.394	.381	0.9	3.1	1.3	0.43	.107	.150	.120	.126
a	16	.278	.016	.351	.088	9.9	4.1	10.9	9.08	.161	.173	.208	.186
c	17	.631	.525	.422	.520	13.9	0.0	9.2	0.49	.204	.145	.092	.134
c	18	.368	.142	.104	.106	3.7	1.4	0.5	0.94	.093	.106	.105	.107
b	19	.002	.397	....	....	0.0	4.4	...	....	.113	.172	....	....
b	20	.308	.151	.060	.172	8.4	1.4	7.7	1.22	.124	.118	.088	.109
c	21	.078	.265	.354	.239	10.3	11.5	9.3	10.02	.078	.063	.076	.074
a	22	.462	.567	.547	.525	3.8	3.8	0.3	2.52	.086	.081	.099	.089
cd	23	.250	.057	.145	.010	4.9	3.4	8.8	6.36	.147	.185	.197	.178
c	24	.380	.406	.184	.296	16.0	13.8	9.5	12.41	.224	.232	.175	.204
cd	25	.006	.071	.232	.059	7.5	1.9	6.0	5.79	.149	.148	.166	.157
a	26	.202	.010	....	....	2.5	0.4	...	....	.123	.122	....	....
c	27	- .280	.057	.428	.100	3 2	3.4	8 6	4.39	.097	.148	.199	.153
e	28	.684	.431	.073	.367	15.7	0.5	1.8	5.63	.234	.117	.113	.149
ec	29	.026	.129	.177	.114	3.0	1.2	0 1	0.94	.109	.127	.125	.122
a	30	.035	.037	.030	.002	3.4	3.5	0 4	2 44	.119	.171	.130	.134
a	31	.032	.123	.219	.124	1.4	6 1	4.1	2.82	.125	.122	.112	.119
Mean: Normal.		29,650	29.621	29.640	29.643	24.65	30.35	26 57	27.04	0 172	0 170	0.156	0.159
Mean: Obsrv'd.		29.614	29.579	29.591	29.593	30 83	35.16	31.60	32.27				

Highest Barometer ......30.210, at 4 p m. on 22nd ⎱ Monthly range
Lowest Barometer.......28.966, at 6 a.m. on 28th ⎰ 1.244 inch.

High'st obsrved temp.... 51 ° 0, at 2 p.m. on 7th ⎱ Monthly range
Lowest registered " 13 2, at a.m. on 21st. ⎰ 37 ° 8

Mean. high'st obs'v'd tem. 36 ° 54, ⎱   Mean. daily range :
Mean. registered minimum 26 58, ⎰   9 ° 96

Greatest daily range, 22 ° 2, from 6 a.m. to 10 p.m. on 17th.

Warmest day, 7th, mean temperature 47 ° 65 ⎱ Difference,
Coldest day, 21st, mean temperature 16 72 ⎰ -   30 ° 93

The "Means" are derived from six observations daily, viz :—at 6 and 8, a.m.; and 2, 4, and 10, p m.

The column headed "Magnet" is an attempt to distinguish the character of each day as regards the frequency or extent of the fluctuations of the Magnetic declination, indicated by the self-registering instruments at Toronto. The classification is to some extent arbitrary, and may require future modification, but has been found tolerably definite as far as applied. It is as follows :

(a) A marked absence of Magnetical disturbance.
(b) Unimportant movements,—not to be called disturbance.
(c) Marked disturbance,—whether shewn by frequency or amount of deviation from the normal curve,—but of no great importance.
(d) A greater degree of disturbance,—lasting more or less the whole day.
(e) Considerable disturbance of the first class.

The day is reckoned from noon to noon. If two letters are placed, the first applies to the earlier the latter to the later part of the trace. Although the declination is particularly referred to,⸴' rarely happens that the same terms are not applicable to the changes of the hrizontal force also.

Toronto, January, 1852.

H. M. Magnetical, Observatory Toronto, C. W.—DECEMBER, 1852.

Elevation above Lake Ontario, 108 feet.

Humidity of Air.				Wind.			Rain: inches	Snow: inches	Weather.
6AM	2PM	10	Mn.	6, A.M.	2, P.M.	10, P.M.			
.82	.70	.82	.80	SW b W	S b W	SW b S	.....	......	Auror. light 4&5 a.m; li't cl'ds dur. day.
89	71	82	83	SW b S	SSW	NE b E	.....	......	Cl'dy at 6&8 a.m; day clear and fine.
89	75	90	85	NNE	NE b E	ENE	1.020	......	Densely overcast : rain'g fr. 9h.50m. pm.
91	93	95	93	E b N	ENE	N b E	0.060	......	Rain'g sl'tly till 2 pm: den. cldd. all day.
94	87	..	..	WNW	W b S	WSW	Inapp.	......	Densely overcast; drizz. rain at 11 pm.
95	91	90	92	S b E	E b S	SSW	inapp.	......	Overcast all day; sh't rain 1 to 3 pm.
90	90	88	90	SW b S	ENE	SSE	0,460	......	Densely overcast; rain'g fr. 2h.40m. pm.
93	63	71	75	S W	WSW	SW b W	.....	......	Clonded; a few clear spaces occasionally.
84	77	86	83	ENE	ESE	ESE	.....	......	Clouded till 4 pm; auroral light fr. 10pm.
88	70	87	80	SW b W	S w b W	Calm	.....	......	Morn'g clear; cloudy fr. 2 pm.
90	72	70	76	N	N b W	W	.....	......	Overcast; very dull, dark day.
87	65	..	..	W b N	WSW	SW b W	.....	0.1	Morn. clear: aft'n cl'dy, sl't snow d. night
80	92	75	83	W	N	NW b W	.....	0.5	Clouded, snowing occasionally dur'g day.
89	97	79	81	NW b N	S b E	SE b E	.....	......	Generally clouded; dull.
81	80	83	82	S	S b W	S b W	.....	......	Clear save a few clds. rd. horizon; fine.
80	88	91	88	E b S	ESE	E b S	0.745	0.2	Snow fr. 11 am; turned to rain at 1pm.
83	85	92	85	S W	WSW	WSW	.....	0 5	Raining till 5 am; auroral light fr 10pm.
81	67	71	75	W S W	W	W b N	.....	inapp.	Densely cl'd'd; sl't snow occas. windy.
81	86	..	..	WSW	SW b W	W b S	.....	......	Densely overcast; very dark dull day.
67	74	83	78	N W	N N W	N	.....	0.8	Overcast, mild; sl't snow fr. 3 to 10 p.m.
89	59	74	76	N b W	N N W	Calm	.....	......	Li'tly overcast 6&8am; occas. sl't showers
75	55	66	67	Calm	SW b S	SE	.....	......	AM cl'ded; gen. clr. N. to 4pm; ni't ov'ct
92	98	94	95	ESE	ESE	E	0.600	inapp.	Overcast, sl't snow at 8am; foggy.
91	83	81	86	NE b N	W b S	WSW	0.010	......	Rain'g sl'tly 6&8am: foggy; occ. showers
84	83	88	86	NW b W	Calm	E b S	.....	6.5	Overcast, constant snow from 8am.
83	75	..	..	NW b N	WSW	WSW	.....	......	Overcast all day; part. of snow occas.
93	78	96	88	N W	E b S	E b S	1.100	1.0	Snow'g fr. N; turned to rain at 5h45m.pm
97	70	71	79	S b E	WSW	W b S	.....	inapp.	Ceased rain'g at 4am; auror. li't at 10 pm.
74	80	85	81	SW	E b S	WSW	.....	0.5	Clouded dull day; part. of snow occas.
79	9	88	83	WSW	S b W	ENE	inapp.	2.0	Snow'g and very sl't rain most of the day.
91	94	89	92	NE b E	NE b E	N b E	.....	8.0	Snowing constantly and heavily all day.
.86	.80	.83	.83	Miles : 5. 60	Miles : 8.10	Miles : 6.47	3.995	20.1	

Sum of the Atmospheric Current in Miles, resolved into the four Cardinal Directions :

North.	West.	South.	East.
1096 30	2228.30	1370.34	1516.54

Mean velocity of the wind—6.54 miles per hour.

Max. velocity—21.3 miles per hour, from 1 to 2 p m. on 28th.

Most windy day—17th : mean velocity—14 14 miles per hour.

Least windy day—10th: mean velocity—2.77 ditto.

Hour of greatest mean velocity—noon: mean velocity—8.37 do,

Hour of least   "   —9 p m. : . do. —5.26 do.

Mean diurnal variation—3.11 miles.

COMPARATIVE TABLE FOR DECEMBER.

Year	Temperature.				Rain.		Snow.		Wind.
	Mean.	Max.	Min.	Range	Days	Inches	Days	Inches.	Mean velocity.
1840	23.28	41.0	4.4	45,4	3	napp	18	not re-gistered.	Miles.
1841	29.67	45.5	2.4	43.1	7	6.600	5		
1842	25.33	40.3	3.8	36.5	3	0.880	17		
1843	30.59	41.1	2.7	38.4	6	1 040	8	8.1	
1844	28.78	48.9	− 0.8	49.7	6	Imp't	6	4.2	
1845	21.49	37.6	2 7	40.3	2	inapp	12	4.7	
1846	27.72	49.2	3.7	45.5	5	1.215	9	6.0	
1847	30.58	50.0	6.6	43.4	7	1.185	8	6 8	4.55
1848	29.65	49.1	0.6	48.5	7	2.750	7	2.5	5.44
1849	26 92	41.3	− 5.2	46.5	5	0.840	12	6.6	6.33
1850	22.55	48.3	− 9.7	58.0	2	0.190	18	1.5	7.40
1851	21.59	43.8	−10.5	54.3	6	1.075	15	.7	7.37
1852	32.27	51.0	13.9	37.1	7	3.995	10	0.1	6,54
Mean	27.03	45.16	0.03	45.13	5.1	1.648	11.2	11.6	6.25

MONTHLY METEOROLOGICAL REGISTER

Latitude, 43 deg. 39.4 min. N.   Longitude, 79 deg. 21.5 min. W

Mgt.	Day	Barom. at tem. of 32 deg.				Temperature of the air.				Tension of Vapour.			
		6, A.M.	2, P.M.	10,P.M.	MEAN	6, A.M	2. P.M	10P.M	MEAN	6, A.M	2, P.M	10P.M.	MEA
bc	1	29.526	29.684	29.784	29.691	23 2	26 9	21.2	23.47	0.110	0.129	0.110	0.114
b	2	.776	.685	.....	.....	23.4	31 4	.....	.....	105	140	...	....
bc	3	.660	.697	.882	.768	26.9	25.4	18 3	22.95	125	117	080	.106
a	4	.915	.914	.937	.921	11 6	18 3	10 9	14 45	069	072	066	.073
c	5	.900	.792	.656	.769	7.1	23.3	18.7	16.03	058	114	083	.086
c	6	.602	.437	.425	.503	25.8	31.2	21.6	27.97	127	149	101	.132
c	7	.482	.615	.768	.637	29.8	38.4	27.2	30 95	143	170	130	.164
cd	8	.794	.706	.604	.696	21.6	36 0	35.0	31.77	101	196	188	.168
cd	9	.578	.723	.....	...	36.3	40.9	.....	.....	197	178	...	....
c	10	.690	.752	.813	.777	24.1	37.4	32.4	32.33	113	177	171	.165
a	11	.892	.950	.976	.948	34.5	33.8	30.7	32.55	169	191	153	.146
c	12	.973	.922	.928	.938	22 3	21.1	17.7	21.08	110	059	088	.086
c	13	.893	.865	.872	.879	20.2	26.0	23.7	23.47	100	084	116	.105
c	14	.856	.810	.816	.830	23.6	58.0	27.3	26.52	116	125	133	.127
a	15	.731	.676	.809	.752	29.1	31 2	10.1	21.40	142	117	058	.117
b	16	.945	.963	.....	....	—66	4.7	....	.....	024	050	...	....
b	17	.910	.807	.637	.784	5.0	18.0	13.9	12.38	0.8	082	070	.067
c	18	.658	.673	.799	.716	14.4	20.2	14 3	17 62	079	081	091	.084
a	19	.891	.890	.839	.869	18.0	24.9	25 9	23.12	084	102	113	.102
ac	20	.694	.462	.528	.557	21.4	32.9	25 8	27.97	113	132	118	.124
b	21	.632	.634	.596	.621	18.7	34.1	27.9	25.67	087	161	135	.122
a	22	.523	.428	.324	.411	19.7	37.0	28.7	28.05	094	167	143	.134
b	23	.050	28.788	.....	....	30.9	34.0	.....	.....	157	185	...	....
b	24	28.665	28.880	29.160	28.922	33.2	29.7	19.4	27.03	167	112	077	.120
b	25	28.889	28.991	29.174	29 036	27 5	13.6	9.7	16.27	145	061	062	.086
a	26	29.550	29.780	29.876	29.768	-0.3	4 0	7.5	3 72	035	046	044	.042
ac	27	30.050	30.180	30.315	30.187	12.7	19.7	10.5	13.72	065	076	057	.065
b	28	30.293	30.220	30.136	30.211	10.0	27.9	21 0	18.25	062	104	093	.084
a	29	30.006	29.630	29.421	29 657	11.1	35.7	33.0	27.47	074	170	171	.140
c	30	29 496	29.687	.....	.....	35.9	29.5	.....	.....	146	094	...	...
b	31	29.600	29.562	29.826	29 666	22.6	38.6	23.4	31.13	105	179	116	.137
M		29.703	29.691	29.727	29.7121	19.88	27.55	21.72	22 98	0.102	0.120	0.107	0.111

Highest Barometer 30.315, at 10 P. M on 27th } Monthly range
Lowest Barometer 28.653, at 4 a m. on 24th }   1.662

Highest Temperature, 40.9, at 2 p. m. on 9th. } Monthly range,
Lowest reg. Temperature, —9.7, at a m. on 16 }   50.6

Mean highest observed temp. 29 ° 04. } Mean daily range:
Mean registered minimum 14 .89 }   14 °.16

Greatest daily range, 40 ° .9, from 2 p.m. on 15th to a m. of 16th.

Warmest day, 11th. Mean temperature, 32 °.55 } Difference,
Coldest day, 26th · Mean temperature, 3 .72 }   28 °.83

12th, 8h. 23m., p.m., brilliant Meteor in South—time of flight fully 2 seconds.

The "Means" are derived from six observations daily, viz:—at 6 and 8, a.m.; and 2, 4, 10, and 12 p. m.

The column headed "Magnet" is an attempt to distinguish the character of each day as regards the frequency or extent of the fluctuations of the Magnetic declination, indicated by the self-registering instruments at Toronto. The classification is to some extent arbitrary, and may require future modification, but has been found tolerably definite as far as applied. It is as follows:—

(*a*) A marked absence of Magnetical disturbance.

(*b*) Unimportant movements,—not to be called disturbance.

(*c*) Marked disturbance,—whether shewn by frequency or amount of deviation from the normal curve,—but of no great importance.

(*d*) A greater degree of disturbance,—but not of long continuance.

(*e*) Considerable disturbance,—lasting more or less the whole day.

(*f*) A magnetical disturbance of the first class.

The day is reckoned from noon to noon. If two letters are placed, the first applies to the earlier the latter to the later part of the trace. Although the declination is particularly referred to, it rarely happens that the same terms are not applicable to the changes of the horizontal force also.

Toronto, February, 1853.

I. M. Magnetical Observatory, Toronto, C. W.—JANUARY, 1853.

Elevation aboue Lake Ontario, 108 feet.

Humidity of air				WIND			Snow,	Ia	WEATHER.
5 AM	2 PM	10	Mn	6 A. M	2 PM	10 P M	Inches	in che	
.85	87	.94	88	N	NW b N	WW b N	....	.....	Densely overcast dull and oomy day,
84	79	.	.	W b S	N E	E b S	.....	.....	Overcast—Mild
87	84	82	83	N E b N	N b E	N b E	.....	.....	Densely overcast Dull day.
89	70	86	82	N b E	N b W	N N W	....	.....	Unclouded, a m. Overcast from 8 p m.
90	88	78	86	N	S W	S W b W	.....	.....	Unclouded a m Afternoon overcast dul.d'rk
84	84	84	84	S W b W	S W	S S W	.....	.....	L'gt pas cl'ds F'nt Auroral l t from md'nt.
87	73	84	84	S W b S	S W b S	S W	.....	.....	Almost unclouded, few passing clouds.
81	93	92	92	N E b N	E b N	E N E	.....	*0.294	Overcast with light haze, foggy and mild.
93	90	..	..	S W b W	W S W	Calm	.....	.....	Densely clouded all day
85	79	94	8	W S W	S S W	S S W	.....	inapp.	Densely overcast, drizzling rain at 4 p.m.
85	64	89	79	N b W	N E	N E	.....	.....	Overcast, mild, dull and dark.
88	45	86	75	N E	E N E	N E	0.4	.....	Densely clouded snowing slightly from 10pm
89	59	88	81	N E	E N E	N E	0.5	.....	Densely clouded, slight snow or sleet all dy.
88	87	88	87	N E b N	N b E	N b E	0.4	.....	Densely clouded, slight snow till 3 p m.
88	67	78	79	S W b W	N W b N	N Wb N	inapp.	...	Clouded till 4 p m. part snow occa'ly n't cl'r
65	85	..	..	N W b N	N W b N	N N W	.....	.....	A m. cle'r & cold few detached cl'ds fr pm
81	84	89	80	W b N	N W	N b E	.....	.....	Few l t detached clouds pas fine clear day.
89	72	88	84	N b E	N W b N	N b W	.....	.....	Mostly clear 4 pm. afterwards densely cl ded
82	75	79	8	N Wb W	N W b W	S W b W	.....	.....	Densely overcast all day. hazy
84	70	82	79	W S W	S W	W b S	.....	.....	Det'chd cl'ds a m. clear & uncl'd from 6 pm.
82	81	88	84	W b S	S S W	S S W	.....	.....	Uncl'a t'l 4pm att'rwds hazy hallo i'd moon
85	77	90	85	S S W	S'S W	S S W	.....	.....	Gen'ly cl'd few cl'r spa's ocas'ly [at mdn't.
92	95	..	.	N N E	E N F	N	4 0	napp.	Overcast sleet & snow f m noon till 9 p m
88	67	71	78	N b W	N W b N	N W b W	2 0	.....	Sno. t'l 9a m af part'ly cl'r w'd hi'h & sq'al
96	7	85	82	S S W	N Wb N	N W	0.	.....	Sl t snow & hsa d'lt t'l 9 am hallo i nd moon
76	81	66	7	N W	W N W	S W b W	.....	.....	Clouded a m n't clear & unc'ld, [tm 11pm.
79	70	77	75	S W b W	W S W	Calm	.....	.....	Lightly overcast, hazy
83	67	81	79	N W b W	S W	S W b S	.....	.....	Clear & uncl'd, fine day and night.
97	8.	91	89	S W b S	S b W	W S W	.....	.....	Li't cl'ds am, cl'r& uncl'd pm [dis.fr 6 50pm
69	57	..	..	N W b W	N W	Calm	.....	.....	Gen cl'r, f t auro l l't 7a m Zodiacal l t very
84	77	73	77	Calm	S b W	E N E	.....	.....	Generally clouded, cl'r spaces occasionally.
86	75	84	82	Mil-s N 5.69	Mile 7.75	Miles, 5 83	7.5	0.290	*A great portion of this was melted snow.

Sum of the Atmospheric Current in miles, resolved into the four Cardinal Directions :

North.	West.	South.	East.
2472 69	1911.13	800 84	1064.17

Mean velocity of the wind—6.34 miles per hour.
Max. velocity—25.3 miles per hour, from 11a m to noon on 25th.
Most windy day, 24th. mean velocity—13.58 miles per hour.
Least windy day—10th: mean velocity—1.40 ditto.
Most windy hour—noon : mean velocity—8 37 ditto
Least windy hour—9 p.m: mean velocity—5 20 ditto.
Mean diurnal variation—3.17 miles.

COMPARATIVE TABLE FOR JANUARY.

Year	TEMPERATURE.				RAIN.		SNOW.		Wind.
	Mean.	Max.	Min.	Range	days	Inches	d'ys	Inches	M'n velocity
									Miles.
1840	17.02	40.6	−13.8	54.4	4	1.395	11	not Reg.	
1841	25.11	41.7	− 4.1	45.8	2	2.140	14		
1842	27.54	45.8	1 3	44.5	5	2.170	9		
1843	28.46	54 4	1.5	52.9	6	4.295	12	14.2	
1844	19.95	45.6	−-7.7	54 3	7	3 005	11	24 9	
1845	26 26	43 0	−3 4	46 4	5	Imper'ft	9	22 7	
1846	26.14	41.2	0.3	40.9	5	2 335	10	6.0	
1847	22.88	42.6	− 2.2	44 8	7	2.135	5	7,5	
1848	27.83	51.5	−1.0	63.5	7	2.245	8	7.1	5.82
1849	18 49	40 1	−15.2	55.3	4	1.175	10	9.2	6.71
1850	29.14	46.3	10 6	35 7	5	1.250	8	5.2	5.80
1851	25.62	43.2	−12.8	56.0	4	1.275	10	7.8	7.69
1852	18.54	37.3	− 7.0	44.3	0	0.000	19	30 9	7.67
1853	22.98	40 9	− 6 6	47.5	1	0.290	6	7.5	6.34
M'n	23.99	43.87	−5.08	48.95	4.4	1.825	10	13.0	6.67

THE TORONTO GENERAL HOSPITAL.

Many rumours having declared the intention of the Government to make some changes in the management of the Toronto Hospital ; it behoves us to watch over this movement, to see that the interests of the Medical profession of this Province do not suffer—and now it appears to us, would be a fitting opportunity to consider what may be the rights, privileges and duties of the Medical profession in regard to it. In adverting to the subject we trust to be guided by a genuine spirit of liberality and progress—while we are firmly resolved to eschew all personalities or crimination, and in seeking the public good, to merge all other feelings.

In considering this matter, the subject would naturally appear to divide itself into several heads.—1st. as to the condition of the present Hospital,—2nd as to the duties of the Hospital Trust,—3rd as regards the appointment of Medical Officers,—4th as respects the duties of the Medical Officers,—5th as to the care and treatment of the Patients,—and 6th as regards the position of the of the Medical Students who resort to Toronto to obtain a knowledge of the profession.

1st. The condition of the present Hospital building, is extremely bad, both old and inefficient: and although capable of containing 75 beds, it is entirely without due and necessary ventilation, while there is no chance of properly heating the building; it is likewise without any of those accommodations considered necessary during sickness—to say nothing of the modern appliances of comfort and utility, now recognized as indispensable in every well regulated Hospital. The building is so ill arranged that it is with difficulty any thing like a proper separation of the patients can be made, and as it is, the women are obliged to occupy the general corridor or passage as a ward, besides which the building leaks extremely, and the toute ensemble is a perfect picture of ruin and decay, that ill accords with the rapid progress of the good city of Toronto. There is not so much as an operating theatre, so that if any capital operation has to be

performed, it must be done in one of the wards, perhaps greatly
to the pain, and possibly to the injury of the other patients.

Again, the bad ventilation and injudicious heating of the
rooms, engenders and maintains a foulness of the air which amounts
almost to positive destruction of the patients enclosed within it,
and is extremely dangerous to the Medical Officers, Students, attendants and others whose duty it is frequently to visit the wards.
We would ask how in the name of common sense could it be otherwise, with perhaps a dozen persons taking medicines, with nothing
but a closed stool to resort to, placed at their bed sides, and at the
same time only a common box stove in the room, perhaps heated
to a temperature of 120 degrees, without any possibility of that
effluvia escaping, except by opening the windows, which of course
cannot be permitted in winter—it must be sure to engender a
bad malaria, and render it deadly powerful; and such is surely the
case, for in many of the wards, with the best efforts of ventilation,
the odour which remains is but too perceptible to the senses, the
very walls being corrupted by it. It is almost impossible for a
patient to escape this noxious influence, as is shown by the constant attacks of the Erisipelas, and other irritating constitutional
complaints that indiscriminately effect them, after residing a short
time in the Hospital, but to end this disagreeable matter,—there
is no doubt but that the building occupied as a General Hospital
in Toronto, is a snare and a delusion, alike to the patient, the
Physician, and the medical student. To the poor patient it is a woeful
deception, for when admitted perhaps for some surgical complaint,
and having obtained all the relief which the present advanced state
of science could afford him—he suddenly finds that he has contracted a far more deadly constitutional complaint from the Hospital
air, and which is even more likely to destroy him ; such is almost
invariably the case, for the most simple variety of disease admitted
into that building, is more or less modified by that deadly miasm.
To the Medical officer it is a constant source of annoyance, perhaps he has treated the patient with the most consummate skill and
science, and he naturally expects to find the legitimate result of
his appropriate treatment, but as the deadly poison received into
the patient's constitution so modifies the result, that it is any thing
but what it was intended, and instead of obtaining a cure, he has
to combat a far worse malady at an enormous disadvantage. To the
Student doubtless it is an extreme delusion—he pays his money
in good faith to the Hospital trust, to gain a knowledge of the rudiments of the art of healing ; he sees his Preceptor adopting a
certain line of practice, a practice doubtless the result of a profound knowledge of the principles of his profession, he is naturally led to expect certain results, but how is he deceived and disap-

pointed, when he beholds the nature of the complaint itself changed
by a deadly invisible agent; in despair he fancies that study and
knowledge are valueless, as regards the prosecution of his profession,
for here he cannot gain a true knowledge of disease, hence he is very
liable to give up his mind to some of the popular medical illusions
of the day, or in despair to yield himself to pleasure and dissipa-
tion, and to waste those opportunities which in after life he will
prize beyond all value.   He certainly has one advantage in the
present Toronto Hospital, he may study the laws of that poison-
ous miasma, and we doubt not, that on the diligent Student it will
make an impression that will never be forgotten.   It is thus clear
that the whole establishment is a marvellous indication of the want
of progress and improvement—it is a disgrace to the city, and ill
accords with the march of the other public departments—the very
appearance of the old building, set at an acute angle with the main
street, plainly indicates the antiquated ideas of the dear old ladies
who superintended the erection of the building, and who from some
peculiar notions, which it far exceeds our finite comprehension to
understand, placed the building north and south, instead of
locating it in a line with its neighbours.   Then again all the necessary outhouses and conveniences about the hospital, are shabby
in the extreme, incomplete, and far below the advanced character
of the age we live in.   If these facts are true, and we are convinced
that no individual can make a visit to the place without being
struck with their reality, a new hospital is certainly demanded, the
interests of suffering humanity requires that the present pestilen-
tial building shall be razed from the ground, and a better and
more appropiate one erected in its stead.   The numerous Medical
Students, have a right to require from the fees that they pay, for a
better opportunity of gaining a true knowledge of the profession,
while the city of Toronto, nay the Province of Canada generally
loudly demand at this important seat of medical instruction, that
the progress of the Medical Profession should be onwards, which
is impossible, without an hospital building, and all the necessary
appliances attached to it, in perfect keeping with all the various
improvements of the age.   That such will be speedily demanded
by all classes of the community we have not a shadow of doubt,
and are convinced that the hospital trust will be forced onwards
in the march of public improvement, although it may be contrary
to their careful and tardy disposition.

2nd. This naturally leads us to consider the duties of the Hospital Trust,—this trust as at present constituted, consists of the
Mayor of Toronto, and the President of the Board of Trade ex-Of-
fico, C. Gamble Esq., John King, M. D., and the Rev. H. J.
Grasett. M. A., appointed by Government; the Hon. C. Widmer,

M.D., and Lucius O'Brien M. D., appointed by the Corporation of Toronto, these exercise an unlimited control over every department of the Hospital, they not only regulate the expenditure agreeable to the supply, but also have the appointment of all the medical officers and servants in the establishment. That the Hospital Trust should have the power over all the Hospital Funds, and regulate carefully and judiciously the expenditure of the establishment, holding a wholesome check over servants and medical officers, we are willing to believe—but that they should have the power to appoint the medical officers, we most strenuously deny; such power should not rest with any corporate body, for it is sure to beget a family compact, which is diametrically opposed to the true interest of the Medical Profession, and is very liable to have a baneful influence over the welfare of the patients, for without some necessary check, incompetency and ignorance will, by favour, often stand in the place of sterling merit, and undoubted talent.

With regard to the Hospital Funds, if the reports we have heard be true, there is little doubt but that the Trust has exhibited great care, and judicious management of the funds and estate belonging to the Toronto Hospital, we believe it could not be otherwise under the watchful eyes of the careful and indefatigable veteran Dr. Widmer, and the judicious management of Mr. Brent who have as we are given to understand, so carefully husbanded the resources that they have some £5,000 on hand. This would be fully sufficient to commence a new Hospital, which we have shown to be absolutely necessary—nay was this fact untrue, the ground on which the old establishment now stands, if properly laid out in building lots, might be made to yield a quit rent of £1000 a year, putting it at the lowest notch. The new Hospital might occupy but a small portion of the land, or might be built upon the block of 6 acres owned by the Trust, situated a little further to the westward, these with the other extensive estate owned by the trust in this city, would surely be sufficient to commence an Hospital consonant with the present condition, and future requirements of the good city of Toronto ; besides which it is pretty certain that the Government would aid and assist in so noble a work, the Corporation of the City of Toronto also would not be behind in finding funds, while the good citizens themselves, never deaf to the calls of suffering humanity, would be ready to add their mite, especially when they were convinced that the whole establishment would be an honour to their city, and a striking indication of their philanthropy. The Hospital Trust must wake up, and a new building be erected, for it must never be said that the Roman Catholic portion, are the only progressive part of the community in this respect, and that they, unaided, will build a magnificent Hotel Dieu, which we are assured is at present in contemplation, the land having been already purchased, and the plans marked out for that purpose.

3rd. Another of the duties appertaining to the Hospital Trust, and which we most unhesitatingly condemn, is the appointment of the Medical Officers by the Board, as leading to favouritism, and inefficiency. We think it is our duty in the name of the whole of the Medical Profession of this Province, solemnly to protest against it, as a decided infringement of their just rights. What right has any man, or corporate body, to sit in judgment upon the Licensed practitioners of this Province. If any properly educated Medical man, being a British subject, has been found fit and capable of practising the profession in this Province, and having passed the Medical Board, has fulfilled the law, and in the eye of the law is perfectly on a par with every licentiate in the Province, except with respect to the date of his License, if so what right has any Board of Trustees to place their ban upon him, and for want of favour and interest, set him without the pale of the only honours and advantages to which the profession is accessible. It is as unjust as it is deliterious to the public good. It is certainly adverse to that liberality and progress which the present Government have long professed to advocate and honour; therefore we have some hopes to see it altered. Rather let every licentiate in his turn have an opportunity of gaining all the honour and improvement which a public Hospital can alone afford. It should be his indisputable right after he has passed the Medical Board, in his turn, when a vacancy should occur, (but in no way interfering with the present incumbents,) to enjoy the privilege if he is willing and able to accept it.—It should be a law, that when a vacancy shall occur among the Medical Officers of the Hospital, an offer of the appointment should be made to the oldest upon the list of licentiates, should he refuse to accept it, the next in his turn should have the offer, until one is found willing to take the onerous duties upon himself; this would be a far fairer method than the present—should it chance that an incapable should obtain the situation, a due and proper system of checks, would soon expose his incapacity, and cause his dismissal or resignation. Should inattention, incapacity or inhumanity be exhibited by the Medical Officer in the performance of his duties, he should be called before the Board of the Hospital Trust, and either admonished or declared unworthy of the situation. For although we would deny the Trust the power of the appointments, as adverse to the public interest, still we would maintain that they should hold the necessary checks, and have the power to dismiss or reprimand, for every dereliction of duty. Let it be remembered, that except the honour of this gratuitous attendance upon the poor, the Medical Officer of the Hospital receives nothing for his mental and bodily labour—to the public it must be a constant source of wonder and surprise, that so much rancour and bad feeling should be displayed between antagonistic medical men, while striving for the honour. There is positively no other reward attached to this appointment, than a facile opportunity of studying his profession, and to do this which is his only gain, every facility which it is in the power of a well built, and well regulated Hospital to afford him, should be at his command properly guarded by a due system of checks, this would alike be beneficial to the poor patient and advantageous to the medical student—while the Medical Officer's progress must be onwards, he must learn from the opportunities placed at his command, or he will soon be compelled to resign, and make room for others more inclined to profit by the advantages of their position.

4th. These facts necessarily bring us to the consideration of the duties of the medical officer ; these are preeminently two-fold: to render all the aid in his power to the poor sufferer committed to his charge, and with kindness and attention to communicate all the practical knowledge of disease he is able to the Medical Students, who have entered to the Hospital for instruction. That these duties may be done with facility, regularity and order, too many medical men should not be attached to the Hospital. Four Medical Officers and two assistants with the house surgeon, in our judgment would be found amply sufficient for an Hospital with one hundred beds. The Medical Officers might divide their duties as Surgeon and Physician. The duties of these medical officers should be to attend the Hospital punctually at the hour of 12 o'-clock, according to their turns of duty. Each should be obliged to inscribe his name and the hour of his arrival, in a book kept for the purpose, at the Hospital, and this should be laid before the Board at their monthly meeting ; if the Hospital rule has not been punctually attended to, and no sufficient excuse offered for absence or delay, due punishment should surely follow; for it must be remembered that time is of vital importance to the Medical Student, when he has numerous lectures to attend to. The Medical Officer should visit and prescribe for the patients which have been allotted to him in the several wards of the Hospital, he should take or cause to be taken, a full and accurate record of the case of each patient daily, in a book the property of the Hospital, which should be preserved in the Library of the Institution, to be considered public property, and to be freely open to every Licentiate of the Province, or any Medical Student belonging to the Hospital; who may study or transcribe the case at their pleasure, and at the termination of every case, the result should be duly recorded, and when death shall have unfortunately occured—it should be the duty of the Medical Officer or of one of the assistants to make a decent morbid examination of the body, so as to ascertain the true cause of death, and this should be truly recorded in the same book, while proper drawings and preparations of the diseased parts should be carefully and scientifically preserved, so as to aid in the description; and these should be placed in a museum attached to the Hospital. If these means were fully and properly carried out, the public would soon be able to discriminate between the truly industrious and talented Physician, and the man who only fills the office to keep his better out. It would ensure a careful and judicious attention to the patient, and give the best promise to the diligent Student, that his precious time would not be wasted in delay—while the opportunity of study here afforded him, if duly appreciated, would open to him, an inestimable fund of practical knowledge. It should be the duty of the assistant Medical Officers, to see all the out patients and to prescribe for them, taking down their cases in a book kept for the purpose, and when any present themselves, that require admission into the Hospital, it should be their duty to admit them to the charge of the Medical Officers of the week, and should it happen that the Medical Officer, from accident or sickness, does not arrive at the time appointed, the assistant should be required to go round the wards, visit and prescribe for his patients, in his absence, so that no neglect or de-lay should occur to the patients. The assistant Medical Officers should also be required to make all chemical and microscopic ex-aminations the cases should demand, and these should be recorded in the case book, and demonstrated to the Students. It should be the duty of the house Surgeon to dispense all medi-cine according to the recorded prescriptions, have full power over all stewards, nurses, labourers, and others belonging to the Hos-pital, and to see to the internal order and arrangement of the whole establishment; it should be his duty to visit the patients twice or more daily, according to the requirements of their com-plaint, and to administer every assistance in his power, during the adsence of the Medical Officers. He should see to the diet of the patients, the due execution of all orders, and the careful attention of the nurses in the administration of the medicines, &c.

5th. With regard to the proper care and treatment of the pa-tients admitted into the Hospital.—The Hospital is intended as a public charity, to afford gratuitous medical assistance to the poor during sickness, so that the moment they enter the establishment they are the recipients of public bounty, and to a certain extent must be considered as public property; they must cheerfully submit to all the rules and ordinances of the Hospital, or be liable to instant removal, it is certain that if a proper spirit be impressed upon these regulations, such only will be ordained as shall be for the patient's good, and the public advantage. If the patient should not be treated with due consideration and attention,—have any fault to find with the medical attendants or any of the pupils or servants, a proper representation of the matter should be made to the Board, who should be empowered to redress all such grievances. A certain number of patients might be admitted who could pay in proportion to their circumstances, but they must in every case be obliged to submit to the rules and regulations of the Hospital; and were not the funds of the Hospital found able to relieve all the claimants for assistance, the wealthy citizens and merchants of Toronto might be solicited to purchase the admission to one or more beds, by an annual payment of a certain sum of money; when by their direction so many patients might be admitted, and treated in the Hospital should their cases require it.

6th. As to the position of the Student.—As soon as an individual has paid his fee for admittance to the Hospital practice, he should have all the advantages the establishment could afford him, in the study of disease and the acquisition of the rudiments of his profession. It should be considered that the State, by means of this public Hospital has a duty to perform in affording the Medical Students every legitimate means of properly acquiring a sufficient knowledge of his profession. The patients should be to him a living book, in which he should be permitted to study under the guidance of his Preceptor, and with due regulations, every phase of injury and disease to which man is liable. The Student should have an opportunity of performing all the minor operations under proper instructors, and should be prepared to assist, as far as is consonant with his amount of knowledge, in the duties of the Hospital. It should be obligatory upon every one of the medical officers to the best of their ability, to explain the several cases to the Students, either at the bed-side of the patient or at some subsequent period, and it should be required that the Students pay all due attention to their preceptors, and strictly conform to all the rules and orders of the Hospital, for if they controvene any of them they should be called up before the Board, and be reprimanded or dismissed, according to the magnitude of the offence.

Such then to our mind are the conditions which would render the Toronto Hospital a source of great public benefit, an undoubted blessing to this community, and to the Province generally. It would afford an establishment an honour to the city of Toronto and worthy the philantrhopy of her citizens. It would do justice to the Medical profession, affording them a just and unprejudiced

opportunity of distinguishing themselves—placing them in a noble field for the study of their profession, and the exercise of their
humanity.　It would prevent the possibility of the minister of the
day, making a trade of the calamities and misfortunes of the poor
patients, by selling the office of medical attendants for parliamen-
tary influence, or family affection, whereby it must be often yielded
up to ignorance and incapacity, a fact alike contrary to the interest
of the profession, the benefit of the Student, and the advantages of
the patient; while it would freely afford to the poorest person
in the community, a certainty of the best medical and surgical advice and assistance, it would form a sure refuge for the poor during
the severity of disease, when totally incapable of caring for himself,
and would produce a noble field for the education of the Professional Students, and training him up to be alike an honour to the
profession, and a benefit to the Province.

　　Having said thus much with regard to the Toronto Hospital,
we do not see why all the hospitals in the province intended for
the admittance and treatment of the poor, and receiving Provincial assistance, should not be placed under similar arrangements,
and would also think the law should embrace the possibility of the
Municipal Council of each county establishing a Public Dispensary
or Hospital in each of their chief towns.　In all towns and villages
in Canada there are many poor who suffer for the want of medical
assistance, or have to throw themselves on the charity of the medical profession, it would be a noble trait in our Municipal institu-
tions that they were careful of human life, willing to relieve the
miseries, ready to hold out the hand of charity to our suffering fellow creatures, and not let the burden fall entirely upon
one class of the community—the Medical Practitioner.

DR. GOADBY'S PAPER ON THE PRESERVATION OF ANIMAL SUBSTANCES. &c. &c.

　　Agreeable with the promise of the former proprietor of the
Upper Canada Journal, we have the pleasure to present the subscribers with a part of Dr. Goadby's manuscript on the mode of
preparing anatomical and physiological preparations, which we
believe will be found extremely interesting and worthy the attention of the amature as well as the Physician.—We extremely regret
that the whole of the promised production will not be forthcoming
in consequence of Dr. Goadby refusing to afford the remainder of
the matter, a circumstance that placed the former proprietor of the
Journal in a most unpleasant position, forcing him to seek the pro-

tection of a Court of Law, so as to prove to the subscribers' that the default in the matter did not rest with himself.

It would appear, that some slight explanation of the matter was due to the subscribers on this occasion. As noticed in a previous number of this Journal, Dr. Goadby in a series of microscopic demonstrations, had greatly interested the Medical Profession in Toronto, several of whom were anxious to possess in print, the Dr's. mode of making and injecting anatomical preparations, also his instruction for the use of the microscope in these matters; the fact was mentioned to Dr. Goadby, and Mr. Plees the printer of the Upper Canada Journal was introduced to him, when Dr. Goadby made the following agreement with Mr. Plees.—Dr. Goadby was to afford matter, and illustrations for 150 pages, and Mr. Plees was to find all material, print and bind the book, giving to Dr. Goadby 100 copies.—Mr. Plees having the privilege to insert the matter in the pages of the Medical Journal, as an original communication. Mr. Plees commenced the work, and printed some 750 copies of a part of it, when Dr. Goadby was assured by some person that he would never receive the promised copies of the work, whereupon Dr. Goadby refused to supply any more matter, and the work could not be proceeded with, so the subscribers to the Medical Journal will thereby be disappointed of a considerable portion of the promised communication.

In offering this explanation, there is no desire to open anew the spirit of private and political rancor which exhibited itself on that occasion : and while we regret that the impulsive character of Dr. Goadby should have been so easily misled, we cannot conclude without declaring that notwithstanding the misunderstanding here evident, we are perfectly ready to acknowledge Dr. Goadby's talent and ability in the peculiar department of science in which he stands preeminent, and to declare from our love to that science, should a similar opportunity offer, we should serve the Dr. with the same disinterested zeal which marked our effort during his residence in Toronto.

We have to acknowledge the receipt of a pamphlet from Dr. Hall, of Montreal, being a series of strictures upon the New Medical Bill introduced into the present session of the Provincial Parliament by Dr. La Terriere, the report of the Committee on the said bill, and a series of questions addressed to Medical Practitioners in Canada East and West. The spirit of the Bill is evidently an attack upon the present incorporation of the Profession in Canada East, and will oblige every Medical Practitioner, whatsoever may be his diplomas or qualifications, to undergo an examination before the Medical Board, prior to obtaining a License to practice his profession in the Province. There appears something very illiberal, and retrogressive in this attempt, and will doubtless have the effect of degrading many a Medical man who has thoroughly studied his profession in other countries, while it places in the hands of the Medical Board a power to annoy and degrade persons, who may be far their superiors in education, and Medical qualifications; so it will tend to prevent the settlement among us of many superiorly qualified Medical practitioners; at the same time we are fully alive to the difficulties which this Bill is intended to remedy, and feel that the indiscriminate admission of Medical practitioners, upon the simple production of a diploma, without due and sufficient guards, is liable to serious objections and susceptible of great abuse.

The following is the proposed Bill.

BILL.

An Act to amend the Law relative to the practice of Physic, Surgery and Midwifery in Lower Canada.

WHEREAS it is inexpedient that any person should obtain a license to practice Physic, Surgery or Midwifery in Lower Canada, without undergoing an examination before the Provincial Medical Board : Be it therefore enacted, &c.,
That the seventh section of the Act passed in the tenth and eleventh years of Her Majesty's Reign, and intituled,—

" *An Act to incorporate the members of the Medical Profession in Lower Canada, and to regulate the study and practice of Physic and Surgery therein*" shall be, and is hereby repealed.
And be it enacted, That for and notwithstanding anything in the said Act, or in the Act amending the same, passed in the twelfth year of Her Majesty's Reign, and intituled, " *An Act to amend the Act to incorporate the Medical Profession in Lower Canada, and to regulate the study and practice of Physic and Surgery therein,*" no person shall, after the passing of this Act, receive a license from the Provincial Medical Board to practice Physic. Surgery or Midwifery in Lower Canada, unless he shall have undergone an examination before the said Board, and obtained a certificate of qualification from the said Board; Provided always, that nothing in this Act shall apply to females practising Midwifery in Lower Canada under the provisions of the Act first above cited ; provided also that any person who shall have served in Her Majesty's Army or Navy, being on half pay, and producing his Diploma or Commission in the Service as such to the Provincial Medical Board, may obtain a License to practice Physic and Surgery without being bound to undergo an examination.

At an early period we propose to return to this subject, and at the present time should feel thankful to any of our readers, if they would inform us what has become of the proposed act of incorporation of the Medical Profession in Canada West; at the present moment, from what with the destruction of the Law and Medical classes of the Toronto University, and the general want of professional confidence ; the medical profession is in a state of chaos that certainly requires some basis on which to found a better aspect of affairs. We would respectfully press upon our Professional brethren a greater unity of action, and more cordial conventional agreement, than at present appears to exist among them, for without such, we cannot expect any beneficial or satisfactory enactments.

In Cancerous disease of the thyroid (usually scyrrhus) the patient being between forty-five and sixty-five years of age, is of great and uniform density and generally painful; it is developed rapidly, and may attain a large size in the course of a few months; it accompanies the larynx in its movements, shortly limits their extent by attaching the organ to the surrounding parts; it occasions great difficulty of deglutition and respiration from an early period to hoarseness, cough, and spasmodic action of the muscles of the larynx, and pains come on and increase in their intensity,—the distress and anxiety of the patient, his sallow complexion and emaciation, marking him out as the subject of a steadily advancing and destructive malady.

In *medullary cancer of the thyroid* the surface of the tumour may be even and tense, or indistinct fluctuation may be perceived, the other characters depending on the steady infiltration of the surrounding textures, distinguishes the disease from other tumours of the same part.

Enchondromatous tumours are to be recognized by their great density, the slowness of their growth, and the absence of any signs of the extension of the affection to the surrounding parts, and of general evidence of the existence of malignant disease.

The diagnosis of *tumours of the neck, not connected with the thyroid body,* is to be established by reference to the general characters which distuinguish them in other situations, every particular of their history and mode of growth having been carefully ascertained as essential points, and sufficient care being exercised in the presence of a quantity of coagulable fluid, in the interior of a cancerous tumour, lead to the belief that it is of a cystic character.

I shall complete this paper by a short consideration of the important question,—*Whether or not fibre is an essential element in the structure of cancer?*

Much difference of opinion still exists as to what are the parts of a cancerous growth which are essential to it. Professor Bennett states that fibres, cells, and a viscous fluid, are the three essential elements of a cancerous formation, Labert regards the cancer-cell as the only distinctive, constant, and essential element, the predominance of one or other of the accidental and secondary elements determining the varieties of form and appearance; yet he regards the fibres as next in point of importance and frequency, and speaks of them in encephaloma as pale, fine, and in a small quantity. Muller says that the fibres of encephaloma are indistinct, and that the fusiform cells are arrested in their development into fibres; whilst Vogel states, that in encephaloma fibrous structures are wholly absent. As has been before remarked, it is excessively difficult to state whether the fibres which are found in many tumours are really cancerous, or whether they belong to the proper structure of the organ in which the tumour has been developed; and consequently, careful examinations of cancerous formations in organs which contain no fibrous tissue in their healthy state, become of extreme importance in leading to a true determination of the mode of developement and actual position of the fibrous element in cancer.

From the examination of cancer of the brain, and of numerous cases of encephaloma, I am led to believe that fibres are by no means invariably to be found in such growths, and that their fibrous element is accessary and non-essential. If this be so, the existence of fibrous tissue in most cancerous structures remains to be accounted for in either of two ways,—viz., by hypertrophy of the normal fibrous tissue of the part, or by a new development of fibre from the recently-diffused blastema,—a development commenced and completed under the influence of the determining energy exercised by the fibrous tissue of the part itself, agreeably to the law of analagous formations. Presuming that the fibrous element of cancer is developed in either of the methods just indicated, the absence in cancer of the brain is readily accounted for, as in that organ there is no fibrous tissue to acquire an unusual development, or to determine the formation of new tissue of its own kind from cells. *If* proper *cancer cells,* of a fusiform shape, *ever become transformed into fibres,* their presence in cancer of the brain, unaccompanied by the fibrous element, may be owing to a deficiency of the stimulus necessary to ensure such development, and may possibly be dependent on the absence of fibres in the original and healthy texture of the organ.— *Monthly Journal of Med. Science,* Dec. 1850, *p.* 523.—(General remarks on the Diagnosis of Tumours of the neck. Continued from the last number.)

ON THE SPECIFIC GRAVITY OF CEREBRAL SUBSTANCE, AND ON ATROPHY OF THE BRAIN.

By John Charles Bucknell, M. D. London.,

Physician to the Devon County Lunatic Asylum.

Hitherto, in pathological description of the cerebral substance, the terms softening and induration have been used in the most loose and uncertain manner When actual ramollissement proceeding to liquefaction occurs, there can be no doubt about the matter, and the senses of touch and sight require no adjuvants. These decided changes are found when limited portions only of the organ are affected ; but when these pathological changes implicate the whole of the brain, death takes place before they have proceeded so far as to leave very sensible and appreciable alterations of structure.

M. Guislain, in his recent work on " Les Phrenopathies," remarks on this subject —" In taking our senses for guides we are liable to deceive ourselves. That which we call ramollissement is only a pathological state arrived at its ' summum' of disorganization ; but does not this disorganization already exist in the intimate structure of the primitive fibres before having attained that visible point of softness which constitutes visible ramollissement ?"

The brain of a patient who has died of delirium tremens, of the delirium of fever, or of some forms of insanity, is not obviously different from that of a man who has been cut off in the midst of health by some sudden accident ; yet we are unavoidably impelled by our casualty to refer the death in the former instances to some change in the brain, which the perfection of our senes prevents us from observing. Perhaps this change is in great measure chemicals; and observations now pending, may succeed in fixing the cause of several morbid conditions of the nervous system on the quantity and state of combination of the phosphorus contained in it.

Perhaps this change is for the most part molecular. The functions of the brain may only be perfected when a certain definite arrangement exists but were its vessels, cells, and tubules, favourable to the regulated passage of the contents of the one into the other, and to the developement and interchange of electrical affinites. This arrangement may be disarranged without addition to or abstraction from, the material of the organ, as in the sudden loss of all function from concussion. Frequent concussion alters the molecular arrangements in the axles of locomotive engines producing brittleness fraught with the most perilous consequences, but giving no external sign that the tough metal has lost its temper. So a blow on the head will kill a man without leaving any change as yet discoverable either by the chemist or microscopist'; perhaps this mystery will hereafter be unveiled to the latter.

I do not believe that the brain is nothing more than a galvanic battery "perfectionated," but the two have so many points in common, that for a long time past a legitimate analogy has been drawn between them. Pursuing this analogy, we find that the working of a galvanatic battery may be impared by the liquid in the cells becoming neutralized, by the disarrangement of the plates, or by interposition of any substance having feeble powers of conduction; on the other hand, the functions of the brain may be impaired or interrupted by an alteration of the nutritive fluid; by a sudden shock which may disarrange the vesicles and tubules; or, thirdly, by the interposition of inert material between its active molecules. It is to this last condition in particular that I am anxious to direct attention.

The interposing material may be albuminous, or fatty, or serous. An albuminous deposit pervading the brain appears to be the condition known as hypertrophy of that organ. This condition is rare. Out of 240 autopsies of insane patients, I have only met with one.

The depositions of fatty material in the brain is a subject of deep importance and interest. In examining circumscribed softenings under the microscope, I have almost invariably found a great increase of fat-globules; but as yet I have been unable to satisfy myself whether, in any changes pervading the whole organ, the fatty material is increased.

The deposition of serous fluid throughout the substance of the organ, is a frequent condition, and is I think, constant in cases of general paralysis, dementia, and all forms of chronic mental disease accompanied by loss of power. Those cases, however, which are occasioned and accompanied by epilepsy, form an exception.

I have long felt the want of some trustworthy measure of the relative amount of the solid and fluid constituents of the brain. The best morbid anatomists have been in the habit of describing the brain as denser, or softer, or more watery than natural, with about as much accuracy as we say the day is cold, when we refer to our own sensations, and not to the indications of the thermometer. We know that these latter sensations often differ in different individuals, to the amount of a great-coat or two; and we may expect that the unassisted senses will not always be very accurate in the former case. If, when examining a diseased brain we could always have a healthy brain before us, as a standard of comparison, we might by the resistance opposed to the knife or to the finger, form a fair approximation to the truth; but facilities for this comparative examination are not often attainable.

For several years past I have sought to meet in some degree the difficulty, by endeavours to ascertain the specific gravity of healthy and diseased brain; and in my annual report, which I presented this time last year, I gave a tabular statement of thiry-two cases in which the specific gravity of the cerebrum and cerebellum, the weight of the brain, and the capacity of the cranial cavity, had been accurately ascertained. I append hereunto a similar table of thirty other cases which I have examined during the current year.

No. in the Admission Book.	Age at Death.	Sex.	Form the Mental Disease when Admitted.	Apparent cause of Death.	Capacity of Cranial Cavity Water 60° F.	Weight of Brain.	Specific Gravity of Cerebrum.	Specific Gravity of Cerebellum.
					oz. (Apoth)	Oz. (Av.)		
933	72	F.	Dementia	Old age and decay	43	34½	1045	1042
628	47	F.	Imbecility	Phthisis	51½	45½	1041	1043
666	48	F.	Melancholia	Chronic gastritis; stricture of phyloric orifice	54	46¼	1041	1042
382	78	F.	Dementia; shaking palsey.	Peritonitis	51	39¼	1040	1043
722	39	M.	General paralysis	Gen,l. paralysis final symptoms, convulsion and coma	50⅞	44	1040	1045
688	75	F.	Chronic mania	Old age and decay	42½	32	1040	1045
452	53	F.	Melancholia	Phthisis	49	48	1044	1014
794		F.	Imbecility (epileptic)	Epilepsy	42½	40	1044	1046
45	52	F.	Imbecility (congenital)	Phthisis	48¾	47	1040	1042
911	29	M.	General paralysis	Gen. paralysis; final symptoms, convulsions and coma	55	46	1040	1043
914	78	M.	Mania (chronic)	Old age and gradual decay	48	41¼	1040	1045
704	43	M.	Idiocy	Cerebral congestion, consequent on erysipelas	47½	47¼	1046	1046
954	31	M.	General paralysis	Gen. paralysis; final symptoms, convulsions and coma.	53½	44¼	1040	1041
977	37	F.	Melancholia	Phthisis	47⅝	45	1040	1045
271	66	M.	Iidiocy (deaf and dumb)	Fatty degeneration of heart and liver	52¾	48	1042	1045
975	56	M.	Melancholia	Chronic gastritis	57½	50¾	1040	1040
288	27	M.	Idiocy	Gangrena oris	51½	52	1040	1045
1034	53	F.	Melancholia (acute)	Chronic gastritis	50⅜	46	1045	1046
1032	50	M.	Dementia	Phthisis	41	40¾	1042	1042
885	62	F.	General paralysis	General paralysis; final symptoms, asthenic	45½	37½	1039	1039
265	69	F.	Mania (chronic)	Disease of heart and lungs and curvate of the spine.	44 6/8	42½	1043	1046
447	33	F.	Monomania	Phthisis	42⅝	42¾	1040	1042
1038	66	M.	Dementia	Pleurisy	46	43	1040	1042
966	62	M.	Mania (chronic)	Apoplexy	53	50½	1043	1045
930	58	F.	Dementia (epilepsy)	Disease of the heart	44½	45	1037	1041
770	57	F.	Dementia	Phthisis, and disease of the heart	40¼	40	1037	1040
871	59	M.	General paralysis	General paralysis; final symptoms, asthenic	54	43	1036	1042
789	24	M.	Edilepsy	Epilepsy	48	47¾	1040	1040
792	42	M.	Dementia, with hemiplegia.	Gradual exhaustation	49	42	1040	1040
1004	45	F.	Melancholia	Softening of the brain (circumscribed)	39¾	43	1041	1042

In commencing these investigations, the unfitness of the hydrostatic balance for the rough purposes of the post-mortem room, led me to think of and adopt the simple expedient thus described in my report : " The specific gravity of the cerebrum and cerebellum is ascertained by immersing a portion of each in a jar of water wherein a sufficient quantity of sulphate of magnesia has been dissolved to raise the density of the fluid to the point required, adding water or a strong solution of the salt until the cerebral mass hangs suspended in the fluid, without any tendency to float or sink ; and then, by testing with the hydrometer, the specific gravity is thus found with great delicacy and facility, a difference of half a degree in the density of the fluid being indicated by the rise or fall of the substance immersed. The soluble salt is chosen for its possessing no stringent or condensing action upon the tissues. In these eight cases (of general paralysis) the average specific gravity of the cerebrum was $1039\frac{1}{2}$; the highest, 1042 ; the lowest, 1038. The avarage of the cerebellum was 1042 ; the highest, 1045 ; the lowest, 1037. This is below the specific gravity of healthy cerebral substance, which may be taken at 1046. The only notice I find of the specific gravity of the brain is in the chemical analysis of M. John, quoted in Mr. Solly's work, and is stated at 1048. Upon these grounds I submit my right to assume, that in general paralysis the density of the brain is diminished."

It is not improbable that this new method of investigating the condition of the cerebrum may lead to important results. Some parts of the organ have a greater density than others ; the figures, however, refer to large pieces of brain containing a fair proportion of vesicular and tubular substance. The cerebellum has generally a higher specific gravity than the cerebrum. In only two out of sixty-two cases has it been lower. In many instances I took the specific gravity of the whole organ, but finding that it was impossible to free so large a mass from air bubbles, I discarded the result as untrustworthy.

A low specific gravity does not necessarily indicate a diminution of cohesion or the commencement of ramollissement, although it points in that direction. A brain might acquire a low specific gravity from an increased quantity of fat-globules in its tissues, while retaining its normal consistance. I believe however that fat tends to accumulate only in softening brain, so that possibly this course of error may not exist ; but it is nevertheless a point of the utmost importance to determine how much of the diminished specific gravity in brain-tissue is to be attributed to the effusion of serum, and how much to the accumulation of fatty matter. This question may be resolved by treating the substance with ether, and by evaporation. I am convinced that in circumscribed softening of the brain (true ramollissement) the low specific gravity is to a great extent owing to the amount of fatty matter deposited. In the last case on the preceding table, the specific gravity of the cerebrum generally was 1041, while that of the softened parts was 1035 ; and, on examination, this pultaceous substance was found pervaded with an immense quantity of fatty matter. The pursuit of these sources of fallacy will open up a new ground for investigation.

Is the serum effused into softening brain imbibed into the vessels, or does it remain interstitial ? M. Guislain, states that " these cells of the fundamental tissues of the grey substance present themselves *ten times larger* than their normal state. In ramollissement the serum escaped from the vessels penetrates the interior of these cellules and provokes their distension. It is a true imbibition." After diligent search with a first-rate instrument, I have been unable to observe these immense vesicles ; and I think that the loss of cohesion in the brain substance would also indicate that for the most part the effused serum remains interstitial.

I have found that in some dieases which occasion a loss of specific gravity of the brain that organ also suffers actual loss of bulk—an actual as distinguished for an interstitial atrophy. The additional fluid which makes the brain light probably goes to make up for interstitial atrophy, but it does not wholly make up for it, and the brain shrinks from its bone-case. This fact is pretty evident of serous effusion into the meshes of the pia mater but I prove it more satisfactorily by pluging the foramina with clay, re-adjusting and luting on the calvarium, with the dura mater attached, and ascertaining the precise quantity of water at 60 ° Fahr. which the empty cranium thus prepared will contain, and by comparing this measurement with the weight of the brain.

In the diseases accompanied by low specific gravity, the absolute weight of the brain, as compared with the capacity of the cranium, is diminished to a greater degree than can be accounted for by loss of specific weight ; and on the other hand ,in epilepsy, apoplexy. and cerebritis, the weight of the brain, as thus compared with capacity of the cranium, exceeds the standard of health.

Professor Sharpey has kindly pointed out to me, that to perfect these comparisons, it is desirable to ascertain the quantity of water which the brain will displace ; this compared with quantity which the cranium will hold, will show the amount of actual atrophy. This plan I now adopt.

I have in this place restricted myself to observations on the brain, reserving to a future occasion some remarks on the specific gravity of other organs. The simple and easily applied hydrostatic test I have described is ex'remely useful in pointing out the early stages of fatty degeneration of the heart liver and kidney ; and with a handful of Epsom or Glauber salts, or even of sugar, and an hydrometer, the morbid anatomist need never be at a loss to decide whether or not this interesting change has taken place in any of these organs.

The cases in the preceding table were all of chronic character ; the specific gravity of the cerebrum ranged from 1036 to 1046. The table I published last year contained a few acute cases, and the specific gravity of the cerebrum ranged from 1036 to 1052.

In the present table the average specific gravity of the cerebrum in 1040·9 ; that of the cerebellum, 1043. In three cases of general paralysis, the closing symptoms being convulsions and coma, the specific gravity of the cerebrum was 1040. In two other cases of the same disease, the closing symptoms being gradual failure of the powers of life the specific gravity was 1036 and 1039. Similar facts in epileptic cases would appear to indicate that the specific gravity of the brain is higher when life has terminated in coma or asphyxia than when it has ended in syncope or asthenia. No. 930, an epiletic patient, died suddenly of syncope from disease of the mitral valves, and the specific gravity of the cerebrum was only 1037. In other cases of epilepsy, with final symptoms compounded of asphyxia and coma, the specific gravity has never been below 1040, and has reached 1049.

In the preceding thirty cases, the average capacity of the cranial cavity for water at 60 ° Fahr. was 48·2 fluid ounces (apoth,) ; the average weight of the brain was 43·8 ounces (avoirds.)

These investigations are as yet too young to fructify into trustworthy deductions; but I think they will establish the existence of two kinds of cerebral atrophy—namely, positive atrophy, and interstitial or relative atrophy, which may or may not be co-existent. By positive atrophy I wish to indicate an actual shrinking of the brain, and by relative atrophy an interstitial change, wherein the active cerebral molecules suffer diminution, and inert materials are deposited. It will be well to restrist the term ramollissement to the circumscribed and decided softening to which it was in the first instance applied. —*London Lancet Feb.* 1853.

PRACTICAL REMARKS ON THE DISEASES OF THE EYE.
By Dr. James Dixon, Esq. F. R. C. S.,
Surgeon to the London Ophthalmic Hospital.

ON SUB-CONJUNCTIVAL DISLOCATION ON THE LENS.

Published accounts of the accident; singular case of vision being retained after extensive injury. Certain parts of the sclerotic are more frequently ruptured than others; causes of this. Prognosis of ruptured globe not necessarily hopeless; treatment.

That the scletoric and choriod should be extensively ruptured the conjunctive remaining uninjured, and that the lens, slipping out through the rent, should become lodged beneath the unbroken conjunctiva, would *à priur* appear a most improbable occurrence. Such accidents, however sometimes come under the notice of ophthalmic surgeons.

The earliest history of the kind with which I am acquinted, is that briefly related by Edmonson, in his "Treatise on the varieties and consequences of Ophthalmia," &c. M'Kenzie, in the first edition of his well-known work, described a case, and in a later edition, illustrated it by a sketch, taken shortly after the injury. Two other cases were seen by him; and Hunt, Middlemore, Van Onsenoort, Francke, Walker, Desmarres, Rivaud-Landreau, Barrier, Pope, France, and Chadwick, have described with more or less detail, similar cases which have fallen under their notice.

I never myself had an opportunity of witnessing sub-conjunctival displacement of the lens until within the last year, during which period two cases have occurred at the Ophthalmic Hospital, Moorfields.

1. The first patient received a blow with a fist, which ruptured the sclerotic above the cornea, and forced out the lens under the conjunctiva at the same spot. The iris was not torn; but after the lens had been removed, and all irritation had subsided, the pupil remained drawn up towards the wound, and vision was limited to mere perception of light.

2. The second patient was struck on the eye with a piece of wood he was chopping. The rupture took place to the inner side of the cornea. The iris was in the same condition as in the preceding case, and vision impaired to almost the same degree.

It was hardly to be expected that an eye, after undergoing such extensive injury as rupture of choroid and sclerotic, with loss of lens, should still retain much sight; and yet a case came under my own observation, in which the organ not only sustained this amount of injury, but *loss of the whole iris* also, without the function of the retain being destroyed. I did not see the patient until eight months after the accident, the precise nature of which could only be deduced from the existing state of the eye. A description of the case was read before the Medico-Chirurgical Society, but was too short to be offered for publication in their Transactions. I therefore subjoin the account, showing the appearnces presented when the patient came under my care.

Maria M'F——,aged forty-nine, received a blow with a fist on the left eye. The lids became much swollen, and she suffered great pain for some weeks; but she had no medical advice until she applied to me eight months after the accident. The cornea was then bright and clear, but all behind was dark, and no iris visible. On raising the upper lid I noticed a very faint bluish mark, about three lines long, just above the upper edge of the cornea. It seemed as if the sclerotic had been divided there, and afterwards repaired by substance rather less opaque than the original structure. Three or four little dots, like particles of black pigment, appeared beneath the conjunctiva, close to the mark in the sclerotic.

The patient kept her hand over the injured eye, finding that otherwise the light dazzeled it and so interfered with her making good use of the sound one. By means of a convex glass I threw light into the eye, to discover what had become of the iris. I could then see into the posterior chamber, and distinctly perceive the surface of the retina : but no vestige of the iris could be discovered. I held a lighted candle before the eye to ascertain the condition of the lens. A single upright image, reflected from the cornea, showed that the iris was also wanting. Vision was limited to the preception of large objects. She could distinguish the form of a sheet of paper, but could not see letters printed on it. I made her look through a magnifying glass : to her surprise she could then make outsome of the larger capitals. I added to the glass a card, perforated by a small hole, and she saw every object distinctly, and read a " brevier'' type. By thesetwo expedients I had temporarily supplied the lost parts of the organ, the glass acting as a crystaline lens, while the perforated card screened the retina in the manner of an iris.

It appears probable, therefore, that the blow *she* received had ruptured the coasts of her eye—perhaps the conjunctive also—a*nd* at the same time,had completely torn the iris from its ciliary attachment ; *both* lens and iris escaping through the wound, and the-rent in the sclerotic afterwards healing up.

The most curious feature in the case is this—that after so extensive an injury the function of the retina was preserved, while the vitreous humour had been so far retained that the figure of the globe was but slightly altered, and its bulk not appreciably diminished.

Some of those who saw this patient, although unable to account in any other way than I had done for the manifest loss both of lens and iris, had difficulty in reconciling my expressed opinion of the nature of the accident with the very faint traces of injury visible in the sclerotic. But an excellent illustration of the extent to which a breach in the coats of an eye may be effaced was afforded by case 1, related above, in which the lens was disclosed under the conjunctiva, and removed from that situation by one of my colleagues ; and yet eight months after the accident the position of the wound in the sclerotic could scarcely be traced, except by a few minute dots of black pigment which had had been carried out with the lens, and become lodged under the conjunctiva. The appearance of this man's sclerotic resembled so closely that of my patient, Maria M'F——, even to the scattered dots of pigment, that to give a drawing to his eye would, in this respect be almost to copy hers.

From the recorded cases of sub-conjunctival dislocation of the lens, it would appear that the point where the sclerotic usually gives way is either *above* the cornea, or to its *inner* side. Among twenty-six patients, I do not find one instance in which the sclerotic has been torn below the cornea or to its outer side; nor have I myself ever observed such to be the case when rupture of the sclerotic, without displacement of the lens, has occurred. Now, as the sclerotic is equally thick and strong at all the points of any circle drawn concentrically to the circumference of the cornea, the rupture, if it were produced by direct violence, would as often occur at one side of the eyeball as on another. But it seems that the sclerotic always gives way under the extreme bending of its fibres, which takes place at the point nearly *opposite* to that which receives the blow; and this is commonly inflicted on the outer, or the lower side of the globe, the inner and upper sides being protected by the prominence of the nose and superciliary ridge.

The prognosis of ruptured globe, with displacement of the lens, and partial or total separation of the iris from its attachments—even if unattended with laceration of the retina, or large extravasations of blood—must of course be unfavourable; and yet the history of recorded cases of this accident shows it to be by no means of so invariably destructive a kind as to deter the surgeon from all hope of doing good. But he must not trust too much to " energetic treatment;" for those cases seem to have done best eventually where there was the least amount of interference with the reparative efforts of Nature, but where the one essential—perfect repose of the injured organ—was secured.

The striking benefit attending the use of mercury in idiopathic inflammations of the eye, has led many persons to believe that it must be as effectual in combating inflammation resulting from violence. But those who in the latter case, employ bleeding and mercurializing, seem to overlook the fact, that when the coats of an eye ball have been divided, Nature's first attempt towards repairing the mischief consists in *increasing not lessening*, the flow of blood to the part. The breach can only be filled up by the organization of material deposited there by the blood : to bring the patient under the influence of mercury diminishes the tendency of such material to become organized, and thus counteracts the very efforts Nature is making to repair the breach. As to " moderating the determination of blood to the part," inasmuch as we have no means of precisely knowing how much blood is necessary to furnish an adequate quantity of reparative material, we may, by bleeding, be depriving Nature of her very material for cure. The blood of one patient is rich in reparative matter, the blood of another is poor. What means have we of appreciating the exact quantity of this matter which, in any given patient, is being carried to the wounded eye ?

All that the surgeon can do when called in to cases of ruptured globe, is to inform himself, as well as he is able, of the habit of the patient, and endeavour to keep his powers as near the standard of very good health as possible. As regards local treatment, the duty of the surgeon consists in maintaining the wounded part *in perfect repose*, both in respect of motion and light. For this purpose it is not sufficient to bandage only the eye which has been wounded. Both eyes must be kept covered, or the movements of the sound one, will of course be accompanied by corresponding movements of the other. A week or ten days is not too long a time for keeping the lids *uninterruptedly* closed, without examining the injured eye. Premature motion, and exposure to light, are almost sure to be followed by irritation and pain.

T

I need hardly add, that in cases of sub-conjunctival displacement of the lens, that body is to be removed, by carefully dividing the conjunctiva covering it. Should the iris have been detached from its connexions, and hang out of the wound, it should be snipped off close to the surface of the globe. These, and all other manipulations which may be found necessary, should of course be performed as much as possible without pressure on the eye-ball; and this evil may be best avoided by letting an assistant hold the lids asunder with specula. By some surgeons it has been recommended to delay the removal of the displaced lens for a few days, to allow time for the breach in the sclerotic to close. This delay would manifestly be improper if the lens were to be the cause of pain. In that case it must be removed at once.

That the state of patient's bowels should be attended to;—that, if restless he should be soothed with such narcotics as experience may have proved suitable to him, or as the surgeon's judgment may suggest;—that the amount of food should be regulated by the vigour of the patient's circulation; and stimulants either given or withheld on the same grounds: all these are points which must be left to the good sense of the surgeon, since no fixed rules can be laid down as applicable to the treatment of all cases.—*London Lancet, Feb.,* 1853.

ON TEMPORARY ALBUMINURIA; MORE PARTICULARLY OCCURRING IN THE COURSE OF CERTAIN FEBRILE OR OTHER ACUTE DISEASES.

By Dr. J. W. Begbie,—Physician to the New Town Dispensary, Edinburgh,&c.

[Dr. Begbie divides his subject into three parts:—*Desquamative Albuminuria* under which head he classes the urine in erysipelas, Asiatic cholera, and scarlatina; *Inflammatory Albuminuria,* under which he places the urine in the dropsy following scarlatina; and *Critical Albuminuria,* in which he considers the urine in pneumonia and certain cases of typhus. In speaking of the first head, he states his belief that in every case of scarlatina, a small amount of albumen would be found on careful examination. This is generally found three or four days after the commencement of desquamation. In examining the urine, both the nitric acid and heat tests should be employed. It should be carefully made for a few days before, and until the process of desquamation is fairly completed. Dr. Begbie believes that after it has once disappeared, it will not return.]

The Microscopic character of the urine, with which the albumen is invariably associated, is the presence of a considerable amount of epithelial, derived from the different parts of the urinary apparatus. Sometimes the entire epithelial lining of the small tubes of the kidney was present, though certainly not frequently. I do not remember to have seen in the urine of simple scarlatina the albuminous or fibrinous casts of the small tubes of the kidney, the appearance of which is so common in the urine of the dropsical affection. Besides epithelium, the urine generally contained amorphous urate of ammonia, sometimes crystalline uric acid; and occasionally, though very rarely, the urine, though examined very soon after micturition, contained crystals of the ammoniaco-magnesian phosphate. In all such there existed a greater than usual amount of epithelium and mucous sediment. It is not uncommon to find octahedral crystals of oxalate of lime in the urine at the same stage of the disease.

The pathological import which the existence of albumen in the urine denotes, is a point on which difference of opinion must still be expected to exist seeing not only how very different are the facts recorded in regard to the occurrence of albumen, but how varying the estimation of the importance be which is awarded to its presence. While many believe its manifestation to be accidental, and of no importance, there are others who conceive it, if at any time accompanied with dropsy, to be its certain prelude. Both of these opinions I have attempted to show are erroneous, and, at least so far as my own observations go, founded on incorrect data. What then is the cause of albumen in the urine in simple scarlatina, and what its pathological import? I conceive it to be as essential a symptom of the disease as is desquamation of the cuticle—to be associated to a certain extent with that desquamation—to be, in fact, the result of a desquamative process, which the mucous membranes in this disease, equally with the skin, are subject to. Granted then, that this desquamation occurs, when such a change is taking place in the epithelial membrane lining the minute tubes of the kidney, the office of the cells composing which is to eliminate from the blood the matters, solid or fluid, which in the normal exercise of the renal function compose the urine, it surely is not surprising that the albumen from the former should, to a slight amount, enter into the latter. Such I believe to be the cause of its occurrence; nor can I regard its presence as indicating any pathological condition, further than the separation of epithelial cells and their passage in the current of the urine. No symptoms referable to any such condition occur, no febrile reaction, no lumbar pain, no non-elimination of urine, no suppression of its wattery parts not even any diminution in its quantity, and with the exception alone of the presence of albumen, no marked alteration in any of its sensible qualities. I have said that this albuminous condition of the urine in scarlatina is associated with the cuticular desquamation, it is so in the time of its occurrence, and so it is also as regards its amount, for I have noticed the albumen in the urine to be greatest in amount and to continue longest, in those cases in which the desquamation had taken place to the greatest extent. In those cases of the urine of which no coagulability has taken place—for my more recent experience has shown me a few such—there has been no marked desquamation, and no direct evidence of any epithelian separation, as shown by examination of the urine. We know that in many cases of scarlatina, especially in those where the eruption, though well-marked has not been brilliant, extensive, or lasting, it is not uncommon for the desquamatic process not to take place at all, at most to a comparatively very slight extent. Such are the cases in which the coagulability of the urine will perhaps not occur. I say *perhaps*, for in some such I have, notwithstanding, found it. I am still, therefore, disposed to regard the temporary albuminuria of scarlatina as probably as frequent in its occurence, and of the same importance as a symptom, as the desquamation of the cuticle.

[In speaking of the urine in Asiatic Cholera, Dr. Begbie remarks upon the suppression of urine as a marked symptom of a return to the proper quantity of that secretion, marking a favourable change in the disease, in many cases of death from cholera, death seems to have been produced from the poison in the blood, producing coma—such as is ordinarily the case where suppression of urine has occurred.

In Erysipelas, though the urine is frequently found albuminous during convalescence, yet it is not so certainly so, as in scarlatina.

Inflammatory Albuminuria.—Under this head Dr. Begbie refers to one example—the dropsical disease following scarlatina—as follows :]

Every one who has paid attention to the condition of the urine in this most interesting affection, must have noticed the great dissimilarity subsisting between its external and other characters, and those of the urine in simple scarlatina; while in the latter, the amount of urine passed except during the continuance of febrile symptoms, is undiminished, one of the most certain forerunners, as it is always the most invariable accompaniment of dropsy, is the excessive reduction of the quantity of urine. This urine when further examined, is found to contain a large amount of albumen; while under the microscope, frequently blood, not unfrequently exudation corpuscles or compound granular cells, always much epithelium, and the fibrinous casts of the renal tubes are recognised. The symptoms which accompany these changes in the urine are generally well-marked, the most prominent, save the dropsy, being a very uneasy, often severe, lumbar pain, and marked febrile excitement, But independent of these general symptoms, it will I think be admitted, that the characters presented by this urine, while they differ from those of the urine in simple scarlatina, indicate also the existence of a much more serious change in the secreting mucous membrane of the kidney, than a merely desquamative one. In order however, to arrive at a correct opinion in regard to the pathological importance of the change undergone in the kidney during the dropsical disease, it is necessary to bear in mind both the symptoms presented by the patient, and the hints afforded by the characters of the altered urine. These taken together give evidence of general febrile excitement, and of renal congestion, inflammation, and exudation. I have examined the urine in many such cases, and have found the albuminous condition much more lasting than in the simple cases, —indeed observations and experience show now pretty plainly that the long continued albuminuria of dropsical scarlatina, may and often does lead imperceptably—insidously it may be—to organic renal disease. In many instances I have found the inflammatory symptoms alluded to, speedily and entirely disappear. I have not seen many cases of the dropsy following scarlatina, which I had watched from the commencement of the primary disease, but I have seen a few, and in all such the dropsical and aggravated symptoms appeared at the time the temporary albuminuria was going on, and were evidently the result of exposure to cold. This variety of albuminuria, then, which I have called inflammatory, may or may not be *temporary*; it is to be feared that not unfrequently neglected, or even unskilfully treated, the affection it accompanies, lays the foundation of permanent renal disease. In most cases however, it is fortunately otherwise, while in nearly all it may be looked upon as, under judicious management, a curable disorder.

[*Critical Albuminuria.*—Several trustworthy observers have noticed the frequent occurrence of albuminuria in pneumonia, and, says Dr. Begbie,]

To this albuminuria I have given the title of Critical Albuminuria, because my data being correct, and my conclusions justifiable, it is to be regarded as an evidence of a critical action, and commencement of a change undergone by a diseased part, before its return to a healthy state. But I can further illustrate this subject by a reference to the changes which occur in typhus ever. I have found albuminuria by no means an uncommon attendant on the convalescence from typhus; not however, nearly so invariable in its occurrence as in scarlatina, or even so common as in pneumonia; so frequent however, as to lead me to examine all cases in which it occurred, and that with very great care. The result has been, that no one of any such cases has, either at the time, or during a considerable period of observation afterwards, afforded the evidence of any organic change in the kidneys; to account for the albumen in the urine.

The albuminuria in the case of typhus appears to me of special interest as occurring much more frequently, if not entirely, in certain cases of typhus. It is in those cases in which we know, or have reason to suspect, that the deposits, have taken place in internal organs, and we find albumen in the urine. Two or three observations of a somewhat different nature have led me to this conclusion; for example, I have found the urine albuminous in cases of abdominal typhus,—that is, in those cases in which we generally find severe diarrhæa as a symptom during life, and deposit in the intestinal glands as the most prominent lesion after death. In several cases of this kind, which proved fatal, I have found albumen in the urine for days before death; and in others, which happily recovered, I have as frequently noticed its occurrence. In both those instances the albumen appeared for the most part, at an advanced period of the disease, at least after the particular symptoms had continued for some time; while in the former, the albuminuria continued up to death; in the latter, in some it disappeared as convalescence was fairly established, and in others it lasted for a longer period. The amount of albumen in these cases, and the other characters with which the coagulability was associated, were exactly as I have described them in the example of pneumonia; and finding the albuminuria to bear a relation to the deposits in internal organs in typhus, I have been led to regard the kidneys as the emunctories by which the morbid matter so deposited to a certain extent is at least removed from the system,—and so doing, to regard the temporary albuminuria of typhus as a critical albuminuria. It is I think, no objection to this view that deposits, such as those referred to, remain in organs for a lengthened period; for firstly, I do not think that we can pretend to limit the period of their removal or disappearance; and I am inclined to believe that when they do so disappear, the urine will very probably contain the ingredients I have noticed; and secondly, the calceous masses found in the spleen, and other organs, accepted as the earthy remains of the deposits spoken of, certainly attests the removal by some channel or other, of the animal matter of which, in their original condition, these deposits were partly composed. This is an interesting subject, and invites further inquiry.—*Monthly Journal of Medical Science*, October, 1852, *p*, 321.

ON THE INFLUENCE EXERTED BY CHRONIC DISEASES UPON THE COMPOSITION OF THE BLOOD.

By MM. Becquerel, and Rodier.

A paper recently read at the Académie des Science, details the results of MM. Becquerel and Rodier's latest hœmatological researches.—1. The majority of chronic diseases and various anti-hygenic circumstances induce an increase or diminution in the three principal elements of the blood—the globules, the fibrine, and the albumen, and this either separately or simultaneously —2. The globules undergo diminution in the course of most chronic diseases of long duration, and especially in organic diseases of the heart, the chronic form of Bright's disease, chlorosis, marsh cachexia, hemorrhages, hæmorrhoidal flux excessive blood-letting the last stages of tubercular disease, and the cancerous diathesis. The same result is observed in those whose food is not sufficient in quantity or reparative power, or who are exposed to insufficient aëration, humidity darkness &c.—3. The albumen of the serum of the blood is diminished in quantity in the third stage of heart dis-, ease, great symptomatic anæmia, the cancerous diathesis, and insufficient alimentation.—4. The fibrine is maintained at its normal proportion, and sometimes increased, in acute scorbutus. It is diminished in chronic scorbutus, as also in the scorbutic condition symptomatic of certain chronic diseases, which is most often and most markedly observed in organic diseases of the heart.—5. In all the above mentioned circumstances, the quantity of water contained in the blood becomes very considerably increased.—6. A diminution of the proportion of globules is especially accompanied by the following phenomena: a colourless state of the skin, palpitations, dyspnœa, a *bruit de soufflet* heard at the base of the heart during its first sound, an intermittent *bruit de soufflet* in the carotids, and a continuous *bruit* in the jugulars.—7. The diminution of the proportion of albumen, even though not very considerable, when it takes place in an acute manner, rapidly gives rise to the production of dropsy, but it requires to be much more considerable when not appearing in the acute form. Considered in a general manner, dropsy is the symptomatic characteristic of a diminished proportion of the albumen of the blood.—8. A diminished proportion of fibrine is manifested by the production of cutaneous or mucous hemorrhages.—9. In anæmia symptomatic of considerable hemorrhage or insufficient alimentation, the charge in the blood is characterised by a diminution of its density, an increase of the water, diminution of globules, a maintenance of the normal proportion, or sometimes a slight diminution of the albumen, and a normal proportion of fibrine.—10. In, chlorosis, which is an entirely distinct affection from anæmia there may be no changes in the blood whatever. When such are present, they consist in a diminution of the proportion of globules, an increase of that of the water, and the normal quantity or an increase of the fibrine.—11. In the acute form of Bright's disease, the fibrine continues normal, and the albumen is diminished. In the chronic form there is a diminution of globules and albumen, and sometimes of fibrine.—12 Most of the dropsies regarded as essential depend upon a diminution of the proportion of albumen and usually originates in a material cause, consisting in a degeneration of the solid or fluid parts of the economy.—13. In diseases of the heart, the blood becomes more and more changed, as they approach the fatal termination. The changes consist in the simultaneous diminution of globules, fibrine, and albumen, and an increase of water.—14. In acute scorbutus, the principles of the blood do not undergo any appreciable modification. In the chronic form the fibrine is notably diminished, while the globules are sometimes considerably increased. In both forms, the increase of the proportion of soda of the blood explains all the circumstances; but it has not yet been demonstrated.—15. The above modifications should influence our theraputical management of these morbid conditions, as each element of the blood is susceptible of special modifications. Thus when the proportion of albumen is diminished, we prescribe cinchona, and a tonic strengthening diet. A diminution of fibrine and an increase of the soda of the blood are to be met by good diet, vegetable acids, and appropriate hygiène; and by the hygienic measures and the exhibition of iron, we combat the diminution of globules. —*L' Union Mèdical*—*Medico-Chirurgical Review July*, 1852, *p.* 256.

ON SOME OF THE PRINCIPAL EFFECTS RESULTING FROM THE DETACHMENT OF FIBRINOUS DEPOSITS FROM THE INTERIOR OF THE HEART, AND THEIR MIXTURE WITH THE CIRCULATING BLOOD.

By Dr. William Senhouse Kirkes.

[The following observations on the above subjects were communicated by Dr. Burrows, to the Royal Medical and Chirurgical Society.]

As an introduction to the Subject, the author observed that it was a clearly established fact, that the fibrinous principle of the blood might under certain circumstances, separate from the circulating fluid, and be deposited within the vascular system, especially on the valves of the heart. The forms of fibrinous concretions to which the following observations especially applied, were, first the masses usually described as Laennec's globular excrescense; and secondly, the granular or warty growths adhering to the valves, and presenting innumerable varieties, from mere granules to large irregular fungous or cauliflower excrescences projecting into the cavities of the heart. These growths, when once formed, whatever might be their origin, were full of peril, and would often remain so, long after the circumstances which give rise to them had passed away. When of large size, or loosely adherent, they might at any time be detached from the valves and conveyed with the circulating blood, until arrested within some arterial canal, which might thus become completely plugged up, and the supply of blood to an important part be suddenly cut off, from which serious if not fatal results would ensue; or smaller masses might be detached, and pass on into arteries of much less size, or even into the capillaries whence congestion, followed by stagnation and coagulation of the blood, and all the consequent changes such coagulated blood is liable to undergo in the living body, would necessarily follow. Many singular morbid appearances observed in internal organs, and not well accounted for, were probably brought about in this manner. Again the masses of fibrine might soften, break up, and discharge the finely granular material resulting from their disintegration into the circulating blood, and, contaminating this fluid, might excite symptoms very similar to those observed in phlebitia, typhus and other analogous blood diseases. Thus the fibrinous material detached from the valves, or any other part of the interior of the heart, might be the cause of serious secondary mischief. The parts of the vascular system in which these transmitted masses of fibrine might be found, would in a great measure, depend whether they were detached from the right or left cavities of the heart. Thus, if from the left, they would pass into the aorta and its subdivisions, and would be arrested in any of the systemic arteries or their ramifications, and especially into those organs which receive large quantities of blood direct from the left side of the heart, as the brain, spleen and kidneys; on the contrary, if escaping from the right cavities, the lungs would necessarily become the primary, if not the exclusive seat of their ultimate deposition.   A division of the subject being thus naturally formed, the author proposes to consider the subject, first, as to the remote effects resulting from the separation of fibrinous deposits from the valves or cavities of the left side, and secondly, as to the corresponding effects produced by the detachment of like deposits from the valves or cavities of the right side of the heart.   The author then proceeded to elucidate the first branch of the subject, in which masses of some magnitude were detached from the left side, and arrested in an arterial channel of notable size.   This pathological fact was illustrated by three cases, in many respects identical; for in each, death appeared to ensue from softening of the brain consequent on obstruction in one of the principal cerebral arteries, by a mass of fibrinous material, apparently detached from the growths on the left valves. The first case was that of a female, aged thirty-four, of pale and delicate aspect. She had suffered from rheumatic pains, and there was a loud systolic murmur heard over the entire cardiac region.   While under treatment for these symptoms, she suddenly fell back as if fainting.   She was found speechless, with partial hemiplegia of the left side, but there was no loss of consciousness ; the hemiplegia increased, involved the face and limbs, and gradually became complete in regard to motion; but sensation remained unimpaired.   These symptoms lasted five days, when she quietly died.   The post-mortem examination developed much congestion of the pia mater, amounting in some places to ecchymosis.   The right corpus striatum was softened to an extreme degree— being reduced to a dirty greyish-white pulp.   In the posterior lobe of the right cerebral hemisphere, was a similar spot of pale softening.   The right middle cerebral artery, just at its commencement, was plugged up by a small nodule of firm whitish, fibrinous-looking substance, not adhering to the wall, but rendering the canal almost impervious.   The vessels of the brain were generally healthy, except a yellow spot or two in the coats of those at the base of the brain. The heart was enlarged ; several broad white patches externally.   The right valves were healthy, so also were the aortal ; but the mitral valve was much diseased, the auricular surface being beset with large warty excrescences of adherent blood-stained fibrine.   The right common iliac artery, about an inch above the origin of its external branch, was blocked up by a firm, pale, laminated coagulum, which extended into the internal iliac.   The pleuræ were adherent in places ; liver and intestinal canal healthy ; spleen large, pale, and soft, and contained a yellowish-white, cheesy substance.   The kidneys were pale, rough and granular ; within the cortex of the right were several large masses of yellow deposit, surrounded by patches of redness.   Death had resulted in this case from the softening of a large portion of the right side of the brain, which the author considered to have arisen from an imperfect supply of blood, consequent on the middle cerebral artery of the same side being obstructed by a plug of fibrine.   The author then discussed the sufficiency of such an obstruction to produce the effects ascribed to it, and he brought forward many examples showing that atrophy and disorganization usually resulted from any circumstance which materially impeded, or entirely cut off, the supply of blood to a part. The author then directed attention to the probable source of the fibrinous plug found in the middle cerebral artery.   The suddenness of the cerebral symptoms rendered it probable that the blocking up of the artery was equally sudden, and not the result of gradual coagulation of the blood within the vessel. The absence of all local mischief in the coats of the artery at the point of obstruction, as well as elsewhere, pointed to some other than local origin for the clot ; and the author, at the time of the examination, formed the opinion, that a part of the fibrinous deposit on the mitral valve had become detached, and carried by the stream of blood, until arrested at the angle whence the middle cerebral proceeded. This explanation suited equally for the plug found in the common iliac ; for it was quite conceivable that portions of the loosely adherent fibrine might be easily detached by the stream of blood washing over the mitral valve, and when once admitted into the circulating current, they would only be arrested by arriving at a vessel too small to allow their transit along its canal. Two other cases were described by the author, possessing many interesting points of resemblance : one, a female, aged twenty-four ; the other, a male of the same age. Both were admitted into the hospital with hemiplegia of the left side ; each had heart disease, indicated by a long systolic murmur. The post-mortem examinations revealed the following morbid appearances common to both :—

Softening of a limited portion of the brain, producing death by hemiplegia ; obliteration of the cerebral artery supplying the softened part ; coagula in one of the iliac arteries ; fibrinous deposits in the kidneys and spleen ; and the presence of fibrinous warty excrescences on the valves of the left side of the heart. So many and such rare features of resemblance could not fail to demonstrate a very close connexion between the several morbid appearances so exactly reproduced in each case. The author believed that these three cases satisfactorily established the two following conclusions—1st, that softening of a portion of the brain, with attendant loss of function, might result from obstruction of a main cerebral artery by the lodgment of a plug of fibrine within its canal ; 2ndly, that the foreign substance thus obstructing the vessel was probably not formed there, but was derived directly from warty growths situated in the left valves of the heart. The author thought it not improbable, although on the absence of direct proof it was but supposition, till further investigation confirmed these facts, that many cases of partial and temporary paralysis suddenly ensuing in one or more limbs of young persons, especially if accompanied with signs of cardiac disease, might be due to interruption of a proper supply of nutriment to the brain by the temporary plugging up of a principal cerebral artery by fibrine, detached from a diseased valve on the left side of the heart. Other arterial branches, besides those of the base of the brain, might arrest these fibrinous deposits derived from the valves of the heart. In case 1 and 2, coagula were found in the iliac and femormal arteries ; and in case 3, in the renal. The author thought that many specimens found in museums, and supposed to illustrate the spontaneous coagulation of the blood, or the deposition of fibrine within a limited portion of an arterial trunk, were probably to be referred to the same cardiac origin, and he illustrated the point by reference to a preparation in the museum of St. Bartholomew's Hospital. The second subject of inquiry consisted of an examination into the effects produced by smaller portions of fibrine detached in a similar manner, but arrested in the minute arterial branches, or even in the capillaries. The author thought that the singular masses of yellow fibrinous substance found in the spleen and kidneys, and other organs

X

and hitherto described as " capillary phlebitis," " metes'a-is," or " fibrinous deposits," were derived from this cause.   Out of twenty-one cases in which the
author had observed these deposits in the spleen and kidneys, or other parts
deriving blood directly from the left side of the heart, in nineteen there was disease of the valves, or of the interior of the left side of the heart.   In fourteen
of these there were fibrinous growths on the surface of the left valves ; in the
remaining five there was simple mention of valvular disease.   The author
thought that the mere fact of so large a number of cases of so-called "capillary
phlebitis" being associated with the presence of fibrinous deposit on the valves
of the heart, suggested a very close relation between the two morbid states.
The author then entered upon the third branch of this part of the subject,
concerning the series of effects which might result from the introduction of fibrinous particles into the circulating blood, manifesting phenomena indicative of the
existence of a morbid poison in that fluid.   A case was related of a youth, aged
fourteen, admitted into the hospital with obscure typhoid symptoms, the surface body of the being covered with petechiæ.   Delirium, with much febrile
prostration, followed ; he became subsequently comatose, and died.   Upon an
examination of the body, the surface was found covered with petechiæ.   The
pia mater was infiltrated with what seemed recently effused blood.   The surface of the brain thus presented a blotchy appearance, amid these spots were
yellow-coloured patches of various sizes ; some were of a greenish yellow hue,
and had the appearance of being smeared over with pus.   The brain was unduly
congested, and ecchymosis was near the surface ; the cerebral arteries and sinuses healthy ; several petchial spots on the surface of the heart, as well as in the
cavities ; and on the auricular surface of the mital valve some white fibrinous
vegetations, very soft and friable ; a like deposit on the aortic valves, with evidence
of ulceration ; several large yellowish blotches extended deep into the substance
of the cortex.   The intestinal mucous surface was covered with petchial spots,
which were apparent also on the mucous membrane of the bladder, pharynx,
œsophagus, stomach, larnyx, and trachea.   The author considered the mystery
of this case cleared up by the post-mortem examination.   The attack had been
ushered in by a severe pain in the right groin, which was rheumatic ; the ensued
rheumatic inflammation of the mitral and aortic valves, with ulceration of the
latter, and deposition of fibrine.   From these deposits portions had probably
separated during life, and were transmitted with the blood to all parts of the
body, and being arrested in the capillary networs and smaller arteries, produced
the various petchial and buff-coloured spots above described.

   The second part of the paper related to the effects which might result from
the detachment of fibrinous deposits from the right valves of the heart.   Reference
was made by the author to a paper on the Formation of Coagula in the Pulmonary
Artery, by Mr. Paget, published in the ' Transactions of the Society,' as well as
to a specimen in the museum of St. Bartholomew's Hospital, in which there was
deposition of fibrine on each of the pulmonary valves, with old coagula filling
many branches of the pulmonary artery.   In this case several large solid, fibrinous masses were found in the substance of the lungs, presenting appearances
not unlike portions of old pulmonary apoplexy.   Lastly, the author recapitulated
the principle points which he was desirous of establishing, viz.,—1st. That
fibrinous concretions in the valves of the heart admit of being readily detatched
during life.   2nd.   That if detatched and transmitted in large masses, they

may suddenly block up a large artery, and thus cut off the supply of blood to an important part; if in smaller masses, they might be arrested by vessels of smaller size, and give rise to various morbid appearances in internal organs; or the particular mingled with the blood might be but the *debris* of softened fibrine, yet with power to produce a poisoned state of the blood, and bringing on typhoid or phlebitic symptoms. 3rdly. That the effects produced and the organ affected wouldbe in a great measure determined by the side of the heart from which the fibrinous material had been detached; if from the right sid, the lungs would bear the brunt of the secondary mischief; but if, as was most commonly the case, the left valves were the source, the mischief would be more widely spread, and might fall on any part, but especially on those organs which were largely and directly supplied with blood from the left side of the heart, as the brain, spleen or kidneys.—*Lancet June* 5, 1842, *p.* 542.

CASE OF DEATH FROM THE FORMATION OF FIBRNOUS CONCERTION IN THE HEART.

By Dr. Walter Carstage, Saddleworth.

[The patient in this case was aged 64. He was attack with erysipelas of the head and face, combined with symptoms of congestion of the liver. From these he gradually recovered, though the system did notseem to regain strength, and the heart's action was very feeble. Five weeks after the first attack he caught a slight cold, and a mild repetition of the erysipelas, and hepetic derangement appeared.]

These symptoms, however, were checked as speedily as before; the appetite returned and digestion seemed to be easily accomplished; and yet, with all these favourable appearances, his strength failed the action of the heart and respiratory movements gradually grew feebler, and at length without any sign of pulmonary, cerebral, or abdominal disease, these asthenic symptoms slowly terminated in death, just eleven weeks after the first commencement of the erysipelatous attack.

Post-mortem.—With the exception of a slight enlargement of the liver, we could find no organ exhibiting structural change. The lungs were perfectly healthy. Upon opening the heart, however, we discover what in my opinion, fully accounts for the gradual dissolution; a fibrinous mass filled both its right cavities, and sent up large and long branches into the pulmonary artery and its ramifications. The concretion was firm and white, and had an attatchment to the walls of the heart.

Remarks—I have but few remarks to make on this interesting case, and I should probably never have thought of publishing it at all, had not my attention been made before the Medical Society of London, by Mr. B. W. Richardson, "On the Fibrinous Element of the Blood," and which have been reported in the columns of 'The Lancet.' I find that in a paper read by Mr. Richardson in November last, he thus observed: "Lastly, in case of asthema, where fibrinous concretions exist in the heart, the very cessation of the act of life may be owing to their presence and gradual increase, the central organ of the circulation becoming literally choked by them." In January, again, the same author briefly alluded to this subject, and produced a pathological specimen which strongly supported his views; and, lastly in the month of March, on exhibiting another heart in which a fibrinous clot was found, he gave more enlarged views on the matter, and threw out the idea, that during those diseases which are known to be attended with an abnormal quantity of fibrine in the blood, it may be that some of the overplus of fibrine is deposited on the elevated structure of the moving heart; and he concluded by saying that, " In all inflammatory cases marked by great super-fibrination of the blood, and which end by what is called sinking, it would be interesting to learn how far similar concretions in the heart may be concerned in bringing about the sinking state."

Now, without wishing to mention the many theoretical points which Mr. Richardson and other physiologists enter into with reference to the formation of fibrine, &c., &c., I cannot but observe, that the case which I have related above affords striking testimony as to the correctness of the opinions from which I have just quoted. My patient had suffered from erysipelas, a disease in which the blood is always super-fibrinized : he sank in the most gradual manner, and the autopsy revealed no cause for the sinking, except (what was surely sufficient) a large fibrinous concretion in the heart.

Of course the narration of a single case does not go far to establish any new opinion, but perhaps it may excite others to turn their attention to the same subject. I have been pzzled, over and over again, at seeing patients gradually sink into death, after some slight disorder, with no evident disease that could account for such a serious result. Now if any explanation so simple as that given by Mr. Richardson should prove after further research, to account for some of these occurrences, a great step in the practice of medicine will certainly have been made.—*Med Times Gazette, Sep.* 11, 1852, *p.* 259.

ON FIBRINOUS DEPOSITS ON THE LINING MEMBRANE OF VEINS.
By Henry Lee, Esq.

Simple inflammation of the veins—that is to say, inflammation commencing in the coast of veins—is regarded by the author as a very rare disease. The lateral lining of veins especially would appear to be as little susceptible of inflammation as any structure in the body. The large number of instances of phlebitis met with in surgical works, occurring in daily practice, are regarded by the author as depending upon and as being excited by, a vitiated condition of the blood. This opinion is principally supported by the two following facts : first, that in every case of so-called inflammation of the veins, the blood will be found to have coagulated in the vessels; and secondly that where such coagulation does not take place, no inflammation will be produced. Continental writers of the highest reputation, have indeed mentioned the concentric layers of lymph which are secreted as the result of inflammation in the interior of veins and English writers, whose names carry with them the greatest authority, have described the adhesions of the opposed sides of the veins by lymph secreted from the capillaries under a state of inflammation. The advocates of this view have particularly referred to an experiment by M. Gendrin in which he mentions that by introducing irritating substances into the arteries and veins, he obtained large deposits of lymph upon their interior. The author on the contrary, having found that inflammation of the coasts of the veins only occurred in cases where the blood has previously coagulated in them, was induced to believe that the deposit found in the veins might be derived directly from the blood. M.

'Gendrin's experiment was therefore repeated, precautions being taken to exclude all blood from the vessels; and it was found that under these circumstances no lymph was effused in the vein. The lining membrane of the veins does not contain any blood-vessels of its own nor does it required any, being in direct contact with the blood. It appears reasonable to suppose, that under such circumstances it would not secrete lymph, and the experiments and observations of the author lead him to this conclusion. The lining membrane of a vein, the outer coats of which are inflamed, may undergo various changes, or may be disintegrated, and cast off into the cavity of the vessels. Lymph and pus may then be secreted into the interior of the canal; but this can only occur in the latter stage of the disease. The readiness with which some morbid poisons produce coagulation of the blood, and the constancy with which such coagulation (indicated by the cord-like induration of the vessels) is found to precede the other symptoms of inflammation, lead to the conclusion, that a vitiated condition of the blood is the common cause of phlebitis. Under such circumstances, although the irritation produced is caused by the morbid matter detained in the vein, yet the inflammation is at first manifest in the surrounding parts. The cellular tissue becomes distended with serum; the cellular coat of the vein then becomes thickened, red and inflamed; and finally, the changes which have been noticed extend to the lining membrane. The effects of inflammation thus are shown to extend to, and not from, the internal surface of veins. M. Cruveilhier indeed regards the coagulation of blood in a vessel as the effect of inflammation previously existing. But the author has satisfied himself, that if blood be prevented from stagnating in a vein, no change will be thereby produced in its lining membrane. The inflammation is not therefore propagated by continuity of surface, as has been generally supposed, but by the stagnation, in different parts of the vitiated blood. Coagulation of the blood would therefore appear to be the cause, and not the effect of inflammation of veins. This view is further supported by the fact, that simple adhesive inflammation of a vein will not produce coagulation of its contents. A preparation was exhibited, showing the effects of a ligature upon a vein tweny-four hours before death. No coagulation of the blood, nor deposits of fibrine on the lining membrane, had in this case taken place. The coats of the vein were thrown into folds, and a white band marked the situation of the ligature: but the projecting folds of the lining membrane presented their natural, smooth, polished, and lubricated appearance. Healthy venous blood will remain fluid for days, when confined in a vein by a ligature. In this respect there is a contrast between a vein and an artery. In the latter case, the internal coats are divided, and the blood coming into contact with the divided edges, immediately coagulates. In the vein, on the contrary, the lining membrane is not divided, therefore the blood remains in contact only with the natural lining of the vessel. Cases in which a small quantity of pus has been introduced into a vein affords the strongest contrast to those in which the coats have been mechanically irritated. In the latter case no coagulum will form, or only sufficient to unite any lesion there may be of the lining membrane. In the former on the contrary, extensive fibrinous plugs will occupy the vessels. These will sometimes occupy the whole diameter of the vein, and become firmly attached to its sides; at other times the outer layers only will become firmly coagulated, and the central ones will remain in a semi-fluid condition. It will sometimes happen that the central portions will be removed, leaving the outer layers attached to the walls of the vessel. The circulation may then be continued through an adventitious cylinder of fibrine. Cases occasionally occur, in which a delicate velvety layer only is deposited on the lining membrane, which remains unaltered in appearance in other parts. The coagula which form in veins will, under such circumstances, lose, in different situations, much of their colouring matter; and it will be observed that the lining membrane of the vein is coloured (from imbibition) in exact proportion to the amount of colouring matter contained in the different parts of the coagula. It will occasionally happen, that portions of the decolourized fibrin will become organized and intimately connected with the sides of the veins, as illustrated in a preparation exhibited to the society. Such layers of fibrin appear constantly to have been mistaken for lymph, the product of inflammation. The extreme readiness with which the blood coagulates from the contact of purulent matter, affords a most important provision for the security of the general system. It appears to depend upon a faculty with which the blood is endowed for its sef preservation. This faculty, although hitherto unacknowledged by physiologists, doubtless exists and is comparable to the preservative sensibility with which every other part of a living being is endowed. When purulent fluid is introduced into a vein, if the coagula are firmly formed, a local inflammation will alone ensue; but, if the morbid matter extends along the vessels, a high degree of constitutional irritation will follow, and the symptoms will occasionally bear a striking resemblance to those of typhus fever. In cases as they present themselves in practice, these two sets of symptoms are constantly present at the time; but they may be produced separately by a very simple experiment: if, for instance, purulent fluid be introduced separately into a vein, and allowed to remain undisturbed, local inflammation only will be set up, which will terminate in the formation an abscess around the vein. The contents of the vein will then become softened, and expelled externally, together with the contents of the abscess But, if the morbid matter be forced forward, in the course of the circulation, no local inflammation will occur, but the symptoms will indicate either the presence of secondary inflammation in some internal part, or of a general contamination of the blood. If the view taken of the origin of inflammation of the veins be correct, it will be evident, that any treatment, to be effectual, must have reference to the first periods of the disease; and that those remedies will most effectually guard the system against the contamination (so much dreaded in this class of cases) which will favour the sequestration of vitiated blood, and tend to localize the disease. The remedies which have been employed to subdue the local inflammation, appear but too often to have done so at the expense of the general system; for, although the local symtoms have become less prominent, fatal mischief has appeared in other parts. In severe cases, those remedies only can be safely employed which tend to preserve the power of the blood, and especially those which increase its coagulating power, as to enable it to separate that portion which has become infected from the general circulation. Bark and opium, together with a nutricious diet are the means which appear to favour these actions upon the due performance of which the safety of the patient depends; while bleeding and calomel, however useful they may be in a case of simple inflammation of the coats of a vein, appear inadmissible when the disease, as generally happens, originates in its contents.—*Med. Times, and Gazette May* 15, 1852 *p.* 503.

ON THE TOPICAL TREATMENT OF ACUTE INFLAMMATION OF THE LARYNX AND TRACHEA.

By Dr. Ebden Watson.

Professor of the Institute of Medicines in Anderson University, &c, Glasgow.

{Dr. Watson first endeavours to explain the modus operandi of a solution of nitrate of silver on an inflamed mucous membrane. He says:]

There is a little experiment, simple, and easily repeated, which is familiar to all who have paid attention to the recent advances made in our knowledge of the inflammatory process, and which presents us with an excellent occasion for observing the action of the solution of nitrate of silver, in the different stages and degrees of that morbid state. I refer to the excitement of inflammation in tho web of a frog's foot stretched out under a microscope. When, for example, a red-hot needle is passed through the web, the following are the phenomena observed:— A spot in the centre of the inflamed part is sphacelated, destroyed by the passage of the needle through it; a circle round the spot is usually found in a state of complete congestion, the vessels being dilated, and the corpuscles almost perfectly stationery within them, and in the part beyond this circle the vessels are not so much dilated, and the stasis of their contents is not so complete. The stream is seen passing slowly away in the collateral circulation of the un-affected parts of the web.

Now these two circles represent two degrees of inflammation, which it is important to distinguish wherever they occur, and, perhaps, especially when the seat of morbid action is the mucous membrane of the larynx or trachea. That part of the web of the frog's foot in which the stasis was complete represents the most intense, or sthenic degree; the other, in which the stasis was not so complete, represents what is usually called the sub-acute, and perhaps chronic, varieties. And the effects of the solution of caustic on each of these parts are markedly and importantly different. In the part which is most intensely inflamed, the solution, in the direct ratio of its strength, increases the stasis of the blood within the vessels. The latter seem to be unable to dilate further, and are, therefore, little changed, but the nitrate of silver acts through the coats upon the blood which they contain by causing its partial coagulation, and, likewise, by withdrawing water from the serum for the crystals of the nitrate which begins partly to form if the solution is strong. In that part of the web, on the other hand, which had been less intensely inflamed, the stimulant solution causes renewed and increased dilatation of the blood-vessels, and the retarded current moves on in them more freely than before; a cure being thus speedily affected if the exciting cause of the inflammation has ceased to act.

That precisely similar degrees of inflammation occur in the mucous membrane of the larynx and trachea with those just described as artificially produced in the frog's foot, I need hardly attempt to prove, for it will be at once admitted that there are three kinds of acute laryngitis; one, in which no false membrane is formed; a second, in which a false membrane is formed, but in which the pharynx, as well as the larynx, is affected, viz., the diptherite of French writers; and, lastly, that intense local inflammation of the larynx and trachea, accompanied by exudation, to which in this country we generally restrict the term "croup."

1. The first kind varies in its intensity from the most trivial catarrhal irritation, to a severe inflammation of the whole thickness of the mucous membrane lining of the windpipe. It very often commences about the fauces and passes downwards, causing cough more or less croupy in its character, difficulty of breathing, and horseness of voice. It is accompanied by fever of greater or less intensity, and its chief physical signs are, in increased loudness of the respiratory sounds in the larynx and trachea, with occasionally a whistling sound, from the absence of the natural mucus of the part, and from partial spasm of the glottis. This kind of laryngitis is more frequently complicated with bronchial inflammation than with pneumonia, and as the patient sinks from non-aeration of the blood, the most prominent symptoms of the laryngeal affection gradually give way, and it is often difficult after death to detect more than a slight redness of the bronchial mucous membrane. The inflammation sometimes, however, terminates in œdema glottidis, and but rarely in the exudation of a false membrane.

I have mentioned the chief features of this kind of laryngitis, first because it is very common in its slightest degree, and is by no means rare, even in its utmost severity; and secondly, because it is not usually a very sthenic disease or, to speak more correctly, it does not present so very high a type of inflammation as that which is characterized by lymphatic effusion, and is, therefore, an example of that degree of this morbid process comparable to the outside circle in the inflamed portion of the frog's foot. The proof of this lies in the absence of exudation.—the usual complication being bronchitis, not pneumonia,—the longer duration of the disease, and its frequent termination in serious effusion into the glottis, or by passing into the chronic form of laryngitis.

It will be expected, then, that the solution of caustic should act well in such cases, and so it does; but pehaps, in none is a greater amount of discrimination necessary in the adaptation of the strength of the solution to the severity of the inflammation which may be present, as well as in choice of the proper time for commencing the topical measures. For it must not be thought that I advocate restriction to any one remedy, local or general, in the treatment of this disease. In the severer forms of the affection especially, depletion of some kind will at first be necessary to check the violence of the inflammation, and, an emetic will be useful in restoring the moisture of the mucous surface. It is after the use of both these remedies that the topical application is alone admissible, nor can it even then be employed to the exclusion of other means. In children it will be especially necessary to repeat the emetic several times during the progress of the case, and in very few will the judicious practitioner refrain from the use of counter-irritation to the outside of the throat while he is proceeding with the topical treatment internally. It is, however, with the latter that I have specially to do at present, and therefore to the management of it I shall, in a great measure, confine my remarks.

Contrary to what might, *a priori*, be expected, the result of those experiments I before alluded to is, that the more intense the degree of inflammation of the laryngeal lining, the weaker ought to be the solution of silver applied to it. In those cases in which the intensity of the inflammation has never been great, or in which, as is more likely to happen, the primary violence of the disease has been subdued by other treatment, a stronger solution may be used with advantage. Its first effect, when thus judiciously applied, will be to coagulate the albuminous film upon the surface of the membrane which has been stripped of its epithelum and thus to cover and protect it. Another, and almost simultaneous effect, is to stimulate the basement membrane to form new epthelium, and to secrete new mucus, and thus the artificial film of coagulated albumen is by-and-by replaced by a more natural covering, and the surface is lubricated by its appropriate moisture. If, then, a renewal of the morbid process could be prevented, a cure would already have been accomplished, but this is seldom or never the case. The good effects of the topical application wear off in a few hours, and the former abnormal phenomena may even in that time have reappeared in nearly equal severity. The treatment must therefore be continued —the touching of the larynx must be repeated frequently for some days, and indeed until all the symptoms of laryngitis have completely disappeared.

In some severe cases of this kind, especially in adults, there is great danger of a chronic thickening of the laryngeal mucous membrane being left behind, and of the voice being thus permanently impaired. It may, therefore, in such cases be a very good precaution to give a little mercury towards the tend of the acute attack ; but whenever the mouth begins to be affected, the topical application of solution of caustic must be stopped: for the laryngea lining, especially at its upper part, is then far too vascular and irritable to bear the touching, and its only effect would be to cause still greater excitement of the part. It is for this reason chiefly, and because I put considerable faith in the topical remedy that I should recommend the mercurialization to be postponed until the termination of the acute stage. After the mercury has had its required effect, it is often a good plan to repeat the topical treatment for a time, when its efficiency will be found very great in restoring the tone of the voice, and fitting the patient to bear a change of his apartment in the first place, and, ere long, removal to the country.

tubes. The exudation, which in these cases occurs after a short stage of intense erysipelatous redness, sometimes in considerable thickness. It is, therefore, in many respects different from the more local, firmly adhering, lymphatic exudation of true croup.

This seems to be a common affection on the Continent, especially in Paris, and also in New York according to Dr. Horace Green, who tells us that a solution of caustic acts admirably as a topical application in such cases. It seldom, however, occurs in this country, at all events in this city, except as an occasional, and happily rare, form of epidemic.

3. True exudative croup is altogether a different disease. It appears in very sthenic conditions of the general system; the blood is invariably rich in fibrine and corpuscles, and the exudation which forms in the larynx and trachea always contains, and is sometimes chiefly composed of, fibrine. It is, moreover, a purely local affection, seizing at once on the larynx or trachea, and confining its chief violence to one or both of these organs. It is, besides, more frequently complicated with pneumonia than with bronchitis—another proof that the degree of inflammation present is very intense, and to be compared with that which exists in the web of the frog's foot around the puncture of the fred-hot needle. And my experience of the effects of the solution of caustic, in cases of croup, justifies this comparison, and confirms the important inference that such treatment is unsuitable for the degree of inflammation present in them; for I have always found the symptoms of congestion in the laryngeal lining, such as pain and difficulty of breathing, increased by the application of even a week solution of nitrate of silver, and the very act of applying the solution is hurtful in these cases; the sponge generally brings away part of the false membrane upon it, and leaves the delicate and highly vascular tissue beneath exposed, and often bleeding. Pain, anxiety, and I fear, increased exudation, and sometimes ulceration, are thus produced, the original disease being thereby aggravated.

To show that I have not been too easily led to these conclusions, and to give force and point to what I believe to be a very important statement, I shall relate the two following cases, which I venture to think interesting in many points of view, and which I have, therefore, selected from my case-book. One of them illustrates the action of the topical application in an adult case, and the other in that of a child.

Case 1.—The subject of this case was a gentleman past the middle period of life, and before the illness which I am going to describe, particularly strong and healthy.

One evening of the winter before last, he was suddenly seized with difficult respiration, tightness in the throat, harsh, dry, whistling cough, and high fever. All the symytoms of croup, indeed, became very soon but too well marked; and, a few hours after the apparent commencement of the attack, the following were the physical signs which presented themselves:—The number of respirations in the minute was much increased, and yet the feeling of oppression on the chest remained unabated, so incomplete was the inflation of the lungs; indeed the respiratory murmur was but feebly heard in the upper parts of the chest, while the bronchial sounds were dry and snoring in their character. In the trachea the inspiration was long, and accompanied by the harsh sound of the air passing along the dry and narrowed tube. A little higher up, and chiefly at the commencement of inspiration, the glottis was heard vibrating so as to occasion a stridulous sound.

When the patient spoke he suffered great pain, and increased feeling of anxiety. His voice was feeble and broken, being at times deeper, and then suddenly slighter, than his ordinary tone.

There could, therefore, be no doubt that this was an instance of acute tracheal croup, accompanied by exudation. It was treated as such, by emetics, purgatives, hot baths, bleeding, antimony, and calomel, with a blister on the trachea, and in the evening I commenced to apply a solution of twenty grains of nitrate of silver in an ounce of water to the interior of the affected organ; but each application gave great pain and uneasiness, and increased the sense of suffocation. The violent fits of coughing which were thus produced undoubtedly occasioned the separation of small portions of the false membrane, but that was no improvement, since the surface thus exposed was tender, unprotected, and often bleeding. I next followed Dr. Horace Green's example, and increased the strength of the solution twofold. This, however, only made matters worse, and indeed the patient himself began to dread the repetition of the proceeding. Still my faith in the remedy was not completely exhausted; I determined, before abandoning the topical treatment altogether, to use a weak solution of the nitrate of silver; I therefore diluted it to ten grains, and ultimately to five grains, in one ounce of water, and yet I was unsuccessful. It was, indeed, too apparent to me that the larynx was not in a state to bear either the stimulant solution, or the presence, for however short a time, of the sponge by which it was applied; I therefore gave up the topical treatment entirely at this time, and used more ordinary measures. The patient was still further depleted, and more decidedly mercurialized. He was likewise frequently blistered during the next month, by the end of which time he was much improved, but still had a good deal of hard, whistling cough, dyspnœ when he moved about, and great pain when he spoke, referred to the glottidean region. The tone of voice was weak, but not unusually hoarse.

The most careful examination of the chest still showed that the lungs were free from disease. The respiratory sounds in the trachea were loud, hash, and dry, and were accompanied by a pretty constant rale, as if there were one or more valvules of exudation matter still adhering to the walls of the trachea. The vibration of the glottis in breathing and coughing was not so free as formerly, indicating a degree of œdema of the organ.

On opening the mouth, the fauces were seen to be red and swollen, and the epiglottis was felt by the finger covered with soft and doughy mucous membrane.

After careful consideration of all these circumstances, it was determined, in consultation with my father, that two caustic issues should be opened, one on each side of the thyroid cartilage; that the iodide of potassium should be administered in decoction of sarsaparilla; and that I should again apply the caustic solution to the interior of the larynx and trachea, now that the inflammation had passed the acute stage. Under this plan of treatment the patient made daily advances towards health, and was soon able to take exercise out of doors wearing a respirator.

The effects of topical treatment during this latter period were as manifestly beneficial as formerly they had been hurtful. The strength of the solution was at first only ten grains to the ounce of water, but was gradually increased to a scruple in the same quantity. After each application the patient found that in a short time his breathing was freer, his cough less frequent, and his voice stronger; but this improvement at first lasted only about forty-eight hours, at the end of which period the application was always renewed with the good effect of sustaining the improvement. By-and-by, however, the intervals were lengthened with impunity; the gentleman spent the summer at the coast, and is now perfectly well.

I think it worth mentioning, in conclusion, that I still see this gentleman occasionally for a feeling of dryness in the throat, which nothing but the stimulent application seems to relieve. This appears to be a very common state of matters after the caustic solution has been applied to the throat for any length of time. Hence I now and again see a number of my old laryngeal patients who have been cured of all their symptoms with the exception of this feeling of dryness, and it is often both intense and annoying. I believe the most of them would disregard it, were it not for the fear of a relapse into their former state, and I therefore encourage them to forget it if possible, and to use such means as rubefacient liniments externally, or some simple gargle. Still it must be confessed that no remedy for this disagreeable feeling is so effectual as the solution of caustic, and if it be not too strong, and if the intervals of its application be not injudiciously short, I do not think its continued use in the cautious manner just indicated will do any injury to the mucous membrane.

But to return from this digression; the case which I have narrated proves, as clearly as any single case can prove, that the topical treatment is unsuitable during the acute stage of exudative croup: and, were it not for the inconvenient length to which it would protract my paper, I could relate many others, the subjects of which were children, and which all go to corroborate the above conclusion. I have in these cases invariably seen good reason to stop the topical treatment if I had begun to use it early in the disease, because I found that it retarded, if it did not prevent, their favourable progress. One of the most marked of the cases to which I allude was the following, and I relate its chief features here, because it is the last case of acute exudative croup in which I have used, or intend to use, the solution of caustic.

Case 2.—The patient was a girl, four or five years old, attended by my friend, Dr. Peter Stewart, of Eglington-street.

This little patient was suddenly seized with symptoms of acute croup, about the middle of last winter. Dr. Stewart was immediately called in, and at once instituted the most judicious measures to check, if possible, the untoward progress of the malady. Among other things he applied a solution of caustic to the pharynx and upper part of the larynx.

Unfortunately, however, as sometimes will and must happen, under the best treatment, the patient's state rapidly became worse, and Dr. Stewart requested a consultation with my father; and a doubt occuring to the former that possibly he might not have passed the probang fair into the larynx, he likewise asked me to see his patient and apply the solution of caustic for him.

The child had been about forty hours ill when I saw her, and was evidently in a most dangerous condition. The exudation was very abundant in the trachea, as evinced by the sharpness of the respiratory sounds heard over it, and by the faintness of the vesicular murmur in the lungs; the glottis, however, vibrated during coughing and speaking, and was therefore, free of œdematous swelling. The pulse was quick but not feeble; the surface of the body was hot and moist, and the face was of a dingy hue, the lips being almost livid.

I introduced the probang, the sponge of which had been moistened with a solution of twenty grains of caustic in an ounce of water, so easily through the rima glottidis, that I feel quite convinced that Dr. Stewart, who is in the daily habit of using this plan of treatment in many other cases, especially in hooping-cough, had likewise reached the seat of disease, and that there had been a fair trial of the topical treatment in this case from the commencement. I repeated the application thrice during my first visit, and Dr. Stewart renewed it again in the evening. At my second visit, next morning, I used a stronger solution, viz., one of forty grains to the ounce of water. After each application the child seemed a little easier, perhaps from the passage being partially cleared by the sponge and by the child's own efforts, but she always became worse in a very short time; and although all the ordinary means had been used during the whole progress of the case, besides the topical measure, still the child's state was evidently becoming very hopeless. The pulse was more rapid, but not as feeble as might have been expected, and the colour of the skin was much more dingy—indeed it was almost livid. The child died that evening, and I regret to add, that no inspection of the body was permitted.

In this case the failure of the topical treatment was far too marked to occur in any one's practice without exciting very serious reflections regarding its employment in the disease of which it was an example, and it led me to look back to my notes of other similar cases, as well as to institute some such experiments as that which I formerly related. The results of these observations and reflections have been to convince me of the total unsuitableness of the treatment in question to acute cases of exudative croup.

But I may here be met with the objection, that if, in my cases of croup, the topical treatment was unsuccessful, a very different result ensued in Dr. Horace Green's cases. This impression, however, will not, on examination, be found to be so correct as many may be inclined to think. Nor is it, in my opinion, detracting from Dr. Green's merit to hold that it consists in having effectually directed attention to the general subject of topical applications to the interior of the larynx rather than in reccommending that treatment in cases of croup.

Dr. Horace Green illustrates his little work on croup by thirteen cases. He may possibly refer to others throughout the work, but these are the only examples fully related, so that they can be judged of independently by the reader ; hence they are carefully numbered so as to permit of easy reference. Of these thirteen cases, two are quoted from Mr. Ryland's work on the larynx, chiefly for the sake of the account given by that author of the morbid appearances after death. In these, of course, the topical treatment was not used, so that the cases which illustrate this treatment given by Dr. Green are reduced to eleven. Nor am I convinced that these were all cases of true exudative croup; nay, I think it is certain they are not; for No. V. was a mere hoarseness, and No. VIII. was a spasmodic affection of the glottis which came and went without any symptom of croup at all. Nos. II., VII., and X., were apparently cases of acute œdema glottidis, leaving only six cases, the symptoms of which resemble those of croup. Even some of these six have more the characters of diphtheritis than of croup ; and in one of them (No. XIII) the affection followed measles. In only four of the six cases was the disease fully developed, and of them one-half died. But, supposing that all the eleven cases related in this book were really cases of croup, more or less severe, I do not think the mortality among them, viz., three deaths in eleven cases, was less than it generally is in the ordinary run of croupy cases occurring in the better ranks of life, and treated in the usual way ; and therefore it follows that Dr. Green's experience, so far as we have it in his work on croup, does not show that his success in the treatment of cases of that disease was increased by his using the topical applications to the interior of the larynx ; for he very properly used other measures as well, and the result has been a mortality not at all less than if he had neglected the topical treatment altogether. I consider it no small corroberation of my opinion, in regard of this point, that M. Trousseau states in the 'Union Medicale' for 1851, No. 100, as one reason for his superior success of late years in the treatment of severe cases of croup, that he has discontinued the application of a strong solution of caustic to the larynx and trachea, which he used formerly to insist upon.

The termination of acute inflammation of the laryngeal mucous membrane, whether that inflammation had been of the simple or of the exudative type, in œdema of its loose subjacent tissue, is an event so remarkable and important that I have reserved until now the few remarks which I wish to make on its topical treatment. I believe that the occurrence of the lesion referred to is by means infrequent, and that it is always attended with imminent danger to the patient's life. The rapidity with which the inflammatory stage sometimes terminates in this manner is sufficiently remarkable to have struck every one who has observed cases of the kind. In some of these it is the result of constitutional debility, however that may have been produced ; while in others it seems referrible to a peculiarity in the nature of the morbid process itself. In the former class of cases it generally arises during the progress of some exhausting disease, such as typhus fever, or towards the end of exudative croup itself, when it is always a formidable and often a fatal complication. And even when it occurs as a more primary disease, the inflammation of the mucous membrane appears to be reduced in intensity by the very occurrence of the serous effusion, although it had previously been even of the exudative type. From what has been formerly stated, then, regarding the action of a solution of caustic applied to a subacutely inflamed mucous membrane, it might, *a priori*, be expected to produce a beneficial effect on the œdematous glottis; and this expectation has been remarkably fulfilled in my experience, as the following instance will sufficiently exemplify.

Case 3.—A young child, of eight months old, had severe hemorrhage from the gums after division of them over the incisor teeth, and in the exhausted state which followed, he caught cold, and became affected with the ordinary symptoms of croup, which were chiefly combatted by an emetic, counter-irritation over the throat and chest, and by repeated small doses of calomel. But very soon the chief, nay, only symptom became that of impeded respiration. The child's efforts during inspiration, the dry, whistling sound which accompanied it in the trachea, the nearly total absence of vesicular murmur in the lungs, and the short expiratory sounds, taken along with the previous state of the little patient, rendered it evident that œdema glottidis had occurred; and if to this it be added that the pulse was feeble, the patient pale and exhausted, and that he could hardly be made to receive nourishment,—his extreme danger will not be questioned.

I introduced the probang down to the glottis, but not through the rima, owing to the swelling of its margins. The strength of the solution used was thirty grains to the ounce of water, and it was applied three or four times at short intervals. The effect was soon apparent. Some coughing, and the expulsion of tough muco-albuminous matter first followed, and then the child became quiet; the breathing was freer, although, of course, there was still considerable obstruction at the glottis. In a few hours, this obstruction seemed to be increasing, and the application of the caustic solution was again renewed in the same way, and with equally favourable results. The calomel was continued, and a warm water enema was administered, after the action of which the child took the breast, and slept for a short time. The future progress of the case was marked by a gradual but steady improvement. The calomel was soon stopped, the bowels were duly regulated, and the topical applicants were persevered in daily for two or three weeks, by the end of which time all obstruction to the breathing, as well as the cough, and even a degree of hoarseness which had latterly been observed, had completely disappeared, and the child's general health rapidly improved.

[In another case of an infant, only two months old, to which Dr. W. was called, the symptoms at first appeared only those of a slight cold, but which gradually assumed a frightful degree of intensity. Dr. Watson touched the glottis with a strong solution of caustic, which assisted in expelling a quantity of ropy mucous and relieved the respiration. After a purgative enema, and a tepid bath, the touching was repeated with manifest improvement; only four or five repetitions were necessary, and the child was well in a few days. Dr. Watson then continues:]

On reviewing the whole subject, then, the following are the principal conclusions to which my observations, experimental and clinical, have conducted me:—

1st. The solution of the nitrate of silver, when applied to an inflamed mucous membrane, acts differently, according to the intensity of the inflammation that may be present; in the asthenic varieties it operates as a stimulant of the capillaries of the part, and likewise of its secreting apparatus, while in the sthenic variety it increases the congestion of the membrane, chiefly by diminishing the fluidity of the blood in its vessels.

2nd. In acute laryngitis, in which there is no false membrane, and probably in diphtheritis, in which there is an albuminous exudation, the local application of solution of caustic, varying in strength inversely in proportion to the intensity of the inflammation, may be employed with more or less speedy benefit.

3rd. During the violence of true exudative croup, the stimulant application to the part affected is injurious, but when the disease begins to yield to antiphlogistic and other treatment, it may assist in the cure.

4th. Œdema glottidis, whether occurring as a primary disease, or as a complication of other morbid states, is always speedily relieved, and in some cases effectually cured, by the application of strong solutions of the nitrate of silver to the œdematous organ.

And 5th. It follows as a corollary, derived partly from the forgoing conclusions, and partly from the results of my experience of the topical treatment communicated to 'The Dublin Quarterly Journal' in November, 1850, that the solution of caustic acts beneficially in only one, viz., in the asthenic variety of laryngeal inflammation : for it matters not whether such has been the original character of the affection (acute but not asthenic cases), or whether it has become so under the combined influence of time and general treatment (chronic cases).—*Dublin Quarterly Journal, August*, 1852, *p.* 48.

ON FATTY ENLARGEMENT OF THE LIVER.
By Prof. Bennett.

Fatty liver is now well known to depend on the secretion of a large quantity of oil, which is stored up in the hepatic cells.   These cells are under such circumstances frequently enlarged, and contain oil varying in amount from a few granules to a large mass, which occupies the whole of their cavities.   Not unfrequently livers, which to the naked eye appear healthy enough, may still be demonstrated with the microscope to contain an unusual number of fat granules, and there can be little doubt that considerable variations may exist in this respect quite compatible with a state of health.   Almost all stall-fed animals that do not labour, possess a large amount of fat in their hepatic cells.   Is is only where the organ is much enlarged, altered in colour, and presses upon neighbouring viscera, that its fatty degeneration can be said to interfere with the vital processes.

In man, fatty degeneration of the liver has been observed to be very common in two kinds of cases—1st, in drunkards ; 2nd, in persons labouring under phthisis pulmonalis.   Drunkards are continually taking alcholic liquids, which abound in carbon, and which being too large in amount to be excreted from the lungs as carbonic acid, and from the liver as bile, is stored up in the latter organ in the form of fat.   In phthisis pulmonalis, the excretory power of the lungs is diminished, and the excess of carbon in the tissues and food is thrown upon the liver to be excreted.   Under these circumstances, it is converted into fat and stored up in that organ.

The manner in which the livers of geese are prepared in Strasburg, is by following a process somewhat similar.   They are confined in close cages, in a heated atmosphere, and largely supplied with food.   Want of excercise and heat diminish the respiratory functions, and cause that of the liver to be disordered, and the result is enlargement of the organ from accumulation of fat. In the case before us, such exactly seems to be the cause of the disease. A man is kept stationary watching a steam-engine, in an elevated temperature, whilst he is consuming his usual food, and exceeding in alcholic drinks.

This view, however, has been objected to on the following grounds:—1st, That the connection between fatty liver and disease of the lungs is not general; 2d, That there is no evidence that a fatty liver does not excrete bile as usual; and 3d, That as a considerable portion of bile is absorbed into the blood to be excreted from the lungs, the liver must be considered as preparing material for these organs. Hence it is argued that it would be a strange compensation if the functions of the liver were to be increased, while that of the lung is diminished by disease (Budd.) But if fatty liver be not always conjoined with diseased lung, it will be found associated with some circumstance which diminishes the function of that organ, in relation to the work it is called upon to perform; for instance, the separation of carbon from the alcoholic fluids taken by the drunkard. Again, want of exercise from various diseases, and especially phthisis, whilst, in order to support the strength, wine and nutritious diet are given liberally, may frequently be seen to be the cause of fatty liver. Further, although it be granted that the liver may in health prepare carbonaceous matters for pulmonary excretion, it must be clear that if the lungs cannot accomplish this function, such matters must be thrown back or retained in the liver, and constitute a powerful cause of fatty degeneration of that organ. On the whole, therefore, we must regard excess of carbonaceous matters in the system, and the diminution of pulmonary action, as the chief cause of derangement in the functions of the liver; a view which has the merit of pointing out to us as remedies a diminished diet, a temperate climate, appropriate exercise, and an endeavour to promote the functions of the lungs and skin.

There is another structural alteration of the liver, which, from the colour and general appearance so like bees' wax it assumes, has been called "waxy," and sometimes "brawny," liver. This disease has been confounded with fatty liver, although an examination of its minute structure will show that the hepatic cells present a very different character. Instead of being enlarged and filled more or less with oil globules, they are colourless, shrunken, and for the most part destitute of contents, while the nucleus has disappeared. The lesion seems to me to be a further stage of the fatty degeneration, in which the oily matter is absorbed, and the cell-walls are left behind and aggregated together; but further researches are required to determine this point.—*Monthly Journal of Medical Science, August,* 1852, *p.* 164.

ON CIRRHOSIS OF THE LIVER.
By Professor Bennett.

This morbid change in the liver consists of hypertrophy of the fibrous element between the lobules of the organ and its subsequent contraction, whereby its volume is diminished, and the secreting cells compressed and atrophied. As a further result the large venous trunks are also compressed, and their commencing ramifications so congested that effusion into, or dropsy of, the peritoneal cavity is induced. The nutmeg liver is an incipient condition of cirrhosis, in which the portal system of vessels in the organ is congested. In both conditions, the hepatic cells are more or less fatty and atrophied. Tne fatty degeneration in nutmeg liver may be seen to commence at the circumference of the lobules, whereas in the advanced stage of cirrhosis, all the cells are more or less diseased, some loaded with fat, and others with yellow pigment. Notwithstanding the great organic changes which are frequently observed in this disease, danger is not so much to be ap prehended from interruptions in the functions of the liver, as from the ascites induced by the constriction of the large abdominal veins, which, by distending the abdomen and compressing the lungs and liver, si?, interferes with those important organs, that death is occasioned.

The treatment in cirrhosis must be purely palliative, and directed to diminishing the ascites, by means of diuretics and diaphoretics. The question of drawing off the fluid by paracentesis is one which may arise, in case the swelling is very great, and the embarrassment to the pulmonary and renal organs, extreme. Even then, although temporary relief may be obtained by the operation, there is every reason to believe that, in the majority of cases, life is in no way prolonged.—*Monthly Journal of Med. Science Aug.*, 1852, *p.* 166.

NEW METHOD OF PERFORMING TRACHEOTOMY.
By Dr. C. GERSON.

For the performance of Tracheotomy, Dr. Gerson has contrived an instrument consisting of three moveable branches, which join at the end, so as to form a sharp point, and can be separated by means of a vice at the other extremity of the cone. By turning the vice from left to right, the branches diverge and form a cone, of which the base is turned towards the wound, and which thus resists the tendency of the cartilages to expel it from the aperture.

In operating, an incision of two or three *centimètres* (four-fifths of an inch to one and one-fifth) is made through the skin, the veins are put aside, and the incision, gradually diminishing in length, is continued until the space between two of the cartilaginous rings can be distinctly felt with the nail of the fore-finger. The trachea is then fixed; and the instrument is glided along the nail of the fore-finger, and is made to penetrate into the space between the rings for about three or four *millimètres* (about one-seventh or one-ninth of an inch). An expansion about a quarter of an inch from the point, prevents the instrument from penetrating too deeply. The instrument being held steadily, the handle of the vice is now turned, and the branches of the instrument caused to diverge. When the opening is sufficiently wide to allow the canula to pass between the branches of the instrument, it is introduced into the trachea. The loss of blood is inconsiderable; and the air escapes with so much force, that it would expel every drop which might be inclined to enter the bronchi.—*London Journal of Medicine, October,* 1852, *p.* 932.

Lightning Source UK Ltd.
Milton Keynes UK
UKHW012022021218
333216UK00014B/2294/P

9 780266 582526